# Are You My Guru?

"I love this book. I love Wendy. As she determinedly searches for physical health (and some bliss on the side), you'll relate to what she eats, why she prays, who she loves—and how she somehow manages to laugh through every challenge. Wendy continues her mission to help women accept and appreciate our bodies. Her hilarious storytelling provides an incredible opportunity for us to empower ourselves around the choices we make, not only to live but to thrive."                                    —Ricki Lake

"If you think that finding faith can't be funny, then you haven't read Wendy Shanker. Her book just might restore your sanity (and is much less fattening than a box of brownies)."
        —Annabelle Gurwitch, coauthor of *You Say Tomato, I Say Shut Up:*
*A Love Story*

"Wendy induces awe for her strength and tenacity. Her wit and positive outlook will inspire many struggling with any illness, whether it be physical or one of the heart. I walked away very satisfied."
        —Crystal Renn, author of *Hungry: A Young Model's Story of*
*Appetite, Ambition, and the Ultimate Embrace of Curves*

"An excellent and entertaining reminder that taking responsibility for one's own health can result in the best medicine."
        —Frank Lipman, MD, author of *Revive: Stop Feeling Spent*
*and Start Living Again*

"A poignant, heartbreaking, and hilarious chronicle of illness and healing."        —Susan Shapiro, author of *Lighting Up* and *Speed Shrinking*

*continued . . .*

"No matter what's ailing you: *Are You My Guru?* will help you feel better. Wendy Shanker strikes just the right balance between Western and alternative medicine."

—Louis J. Aronne, MD, FACP, clinical professor of medicine, Weill-Cornell Medical College

"You can't flip a channel, swing a stethoscope, or shop for ground flax seed without encountering an expert—degreed, self-styled or divinely enlightened—who professes to have the answers. And it doesn't hurt to listen. But Shanker's message—that YOU are the ultimate authority on you—is one we'd be fools not to apply to any situation where our health and/or happiness is at stake. Shanker's delivery— earned gallows humor mixed with honest appreciation for even the rawest of deals, sprinkled with pop-culture sugar to make it go down easy—renders her story of changing her posture in life in light of a life-changing illness too intensely entertaining to put down."

—Stephanie Dolgoff, author of *My Formerly Hot Life: Dispatches from Just the Other Side of Young*

PRAISE FOR

# The Fat Girl's Guide to Life

"A brave, funny, empowering, funny, necessary (and did I mention funny?) book. *The Fat Girl's Guide to Life* is chicken soup for the big girl's soul."

—Jennifer Weiner

"Funny, feminist, fat, friendly, and fierce. It's food. It's fulfilling."

—Eve Ensler, author of *The Vagina Monologues*

# ARE YOU MY Guru?

## HOW MEDICINE, MEDITATION & MADONNA SAVED MY LIFE

### Wendy Shanker

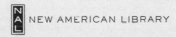

NEW AMERICAN LIBRARY

New American Library
Published by New American Library, a division of
Penguin Group (USA) Inc., 375 Hudson Street,
New York, New York 10014, USA
Penguin Group (Canada), 90 Eglinton Avenue East, Suite 700, Toronto,
Ontario M4P 2Y3, Canada (a division of Pearson Penguin Canada Inc.)
Penguin Books Ltd., 80 Strand, London WC2R 0RL, England
Penguin Ireland, 25 St. Stephen's Green, Dublin 2,
Ireland (a division of Penguin Books Ltd.)
Penguin Group (Australia), 250 Camberwell Road, Camberwell, Victoria 3124,
Australia (a division of Pearson Australia Group Pty. Ltd.)
Penguin Books India Pvt. Ltd., 11 Community Centre, Panchsheel Park,
New Delhi - 110 017, India
Penguin Group (NZ), 67 Apollo Drive, Rosedale, North Shore 0632,
New Zealand (a division of Pearson New Zealand Ltd.)
Penguin Books (South Africa) (Pty.) Ltd., 24 Sturdee Avenue,
Rosebank, Johannesburg 2196, South Africa

Penguin Books Ltd., Registered Offices:
80 Strand, London WC2R 0RL, England

First published by New American Library,
a division of Penguin Group (USA) Inc.

First Printing, September 2010
10  9  8  7  6  5  4  3  2  1

*Author copyrights and permissions appear on page 292.*

Portions of this title appreared in the March 2007 issue of *Self* magazine.

 REGISTERED TRADEMARK—MARCA REGISTRADA

LIBRARY OF CONGRESS CATALOGING-IN-PUBLICATION DATA:

Shanker, Wendy, 1971–
Are you my guru?: how medicine, meditation & Madonna saved my life/Wendy Shanker.
p.   cm.
ISBN 978-0-451-22994-6
1. Shanker, Wendy, 1971–   2. Shanker, Wendy, 1971—Health.   3. Wegener's granulomatosis—
Patients—Biography.   4. Wegener's granulomatosis—Treatment—Case studies.   5. Liver—
Diseases—Case studies.   6. Meditation—Therapeutic use—Case studies.   7. Healing—
Case studies.   8. Madonna, 1958—Influence.   9. Women—New York (State)—New York—
Biography.   10. New York (N. Y.)—Biography.   I. Title.
RC694.5.153S53 2010
362.196'3620092—dc22          2010016228
[B]

Set in Goudy Old Style
Designed by Jennifer Daddio

Printed in the United States of America

PUBLISHER'S NOTE
Penguin is committed to publishing works of quality and integrity. In that spirit, we are proud to offer
this book to our readers; however the story, the experiences and the words are the author's alone.
While the author has made every effort to provide accurate telephone numbers and Internet addresses at
the time of publication, neither the publisher nor the author assumes any responsibility for errors, or for
changes that occur after publication. Further, publisher does not have any control over and does not
assume any responsibility for author or third-party Web sites or their content.

*To Tracy & Sam*

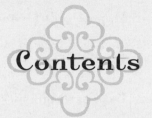

# Contents

CONTENTS

We of the postfeminist generation grew up being told we could do anything, be anything, if we just put our minds to it. Yet, if we have the power to create our own fates, wouldn't the corollary be that we're also responsible for our own misfortunes? And, in a kind of double magical thinking, shouldn't we be able to cure ourselves using the same indefatigable will?

—Peggy Orenstein, "Stress Test,"
*The New York Times Magazine*, December 28, 2008

# Who's That Girl?

madonna has a *sick* body.

She lured me in with the sensual softness of her "Like a Virgin" phase; inspired me with the provocative androgyny of the "Express Yourself" era; and impressed me with the firm ballet-barre derriere of her "Dance Floor" days. Today her every muscle is defined with such intensity that her veins look like long ropes of licorice. She wears that little red string on her left wrist rain or shine, sweat or video shoot, to represent her connection to the Jewish mystical study of Kabbalah. Yeah, I think she looks a little extreme, but I wouldn't mind being in such fantastic shape that I could tour the world with a two-hour dance fest at the age of fifty. Madonna outswivels Beyoncé, and that's no easy task.

Every body tells a story. Here's my quickie interpretation of Madonna's: The longer she's been around, the more shit she has to take, the tougher her skin gets. Her body has become a missile-defense shield against criticism. At the same time, she's a weapon. She looks like she could crush your head between her thighs while she's prancing around singing "Holiday." You don't mess with Madonna. To me, she is an example of unrelenting strength.

I also have a *sick* body. Not fabulous like Madonna's; I mean, literally sick. In 1999, I was diagnosed with a rare, vascular auto-immune disease called Wegener's granulomatosis. At the end of 2003, it flared like Russell Crowe in a hotel lobby. Wegener's caused my immune system to work overtime, fighting an invader that wasn't there. No one is certain how one contracts vascular autoimmune diseases, which include lupus, scleroderma, and hyperthyroiditis, and no one knows how to cure them. Doctors treat serious autoimmune diseases like they do cancer, with a combination of steroids and chemotherapy, hoping to crash and burn the system into a long-lasting remission. There are 50 million Americans living with autoimmune diseases, and more than 75 percent are women.[*] One in nine women of childbearing years develops an autoimmune disorder. To give you some perspective, one in sixty-nine women below the age of fifty is diagnosed with breast cancer.[†]

Cancer is an outside invader your immune system must fight; Wegener's is created by your system itself. If cancer is a playground bully you have to stand up to and fight, autoimmune disease behaves more like the mean girl in the school cafeteria. Mysterious. Nefarious. Insidious. She has no reason to pick on you, but she subtly does her dirty work, tricking your super-well-behaved-up-to-this-point immune system into attacking some innocent cells that were just hanging out with their innocent cell friends. You

---

[*] American Autoimmune Related Diseases Association.
[†] Ibid., p. xvii.

get sicker and more unsure of yourself and your body. By then, it's too late. *You* become what's wrong with you. If you don't get better, there's no one to blame but you. Autoimmune disease feels like a bout of low self-esteem that's gone completely off the rails; it's awful hard to love and accept yourself when it's you you're fighting. It's even tougher to trust yourself to make the right treatment decisions. On top of that, for many of us women our bodies have gone through so much diet drama that we no longer know how to listen and respond in a rational way.

If *autoimmune* means that your body starts working against you, then I say fat is the ultimate autoimmune issue. Being fat and being sick have a lot of similarities. In both cases, my body was doing something I didn't want it to do (gaining weight/screwing up my immune system). I tried everything I could to make it change (lose weight/get healthy). I was willing to go to any lengths, spend any amount of money, listen to anyone who might have the answer. When I failed (to get thin/get better), I felt like it was my fault. I clearly didn't want it badly enough. I didn't love myself enough. If only I had the willpower to triumph over this one problem (fat/sick), the rest of my life would fall into place.

After an insane number of false starts and one particularly dehumanizing experience at the Duke Diet & Fitness Center, I realized I wasn't gonna get skinny. Lack of willpower was not the problem. The body I was born with was the one I had, and if I couldn't love it, at least I could learn to live with it. So I wrote a book, *The Fat Girl's Guide to Life*, hoping the story of my experience could be therapeutic for other women. My body's story had a happy ending.

Just when I had a completely new and well-deserved outlook about myself, *finally* some major appreciation for my beauty and my body, Wegener's struck. The power I felt over my appearance, the control I'd worked so hard to earn, completely slipped away due to illness, treatment of that illness, and one seriously messed-up liver. I had the positive image thing *locked down,* and suddenly I'm inside, looking out of some other body, going, "What the hell happened?" I found it enormously rude that higher powers—let alone my own immune system—had compromised my newly discovered beauty and my recently discovered pride by taking away my health and my looks. So a body battle that I thought I'd won started again, a different fight on the same battlefield. I turned to doctors, then healers, and more than once to Madonna for strength and support. Turns out, the story of my body had a sequel. Here it is.

# Human Nature

DECEMBER 6, 1998

MY 27TH BIRTHDAY

CURRENT FAVORITE TV SHOW:
*Buffy the Vampire Slayer*

CURRENT FAVORITE MOVIE:
*Rushmore*

CURRENT LOOK:
*Wide leg trousers, V-neck top, black boots,
black bob, red nails, red lips*

CURRENT WEIGHT:
*244*

IN MADONNA NEWS:
*Kabbalah-inspired album* Ray of Light *on its way to
quadruple-platinum status. Om shanti, people!*

**B**irthdays blow. Oh, they were fine when I was a kid, and my Sweet Sixteen, if not MTV-worthy, was certainly something special. After a beautiful luncheon and a dessert of warm chocolate brownies topped with ice cream (if anyone ever comes up with a better dessert, let me know), my parents introduced me to my amazing sixteenth-birthday gift: a white 1988 Ford Taurus with a red interior, Michigan plates 835 TUX.

By the time I was seventeen, though, I was doing some uncomfortable Death Math in my head. I became convinced that I would never see the far side of thirty-five, and I was now at the halfway point between zero and the end of my life (I only got, like, 420 on the math SAT, so don't quote me on that). I had a rational explanation for this irrational thought. My mom died when she was thirty-five. Per psychiatric circles, many kids who lose a parent don't believe they'll outlive the age of their parent's death. I tried not to share my concerns about early mortality because a) it tends to bum people out, and b) there wasn't much I could do about it. I'd just have to wait out the next seventeen years or so and see if I was right.

On my ticking Life Clock, my twenty-seventh birthday left me with a balance of eight years to go, cheerfully waiting for cancer to pop up or a bus to slam into me. Even for people without a not-death wish, there's nothing significant about a twenty-seventh birthday. Since I'm a December baby, my birthday usually gets rolled into Christmas and Hanukkah and New Year's anyway. Fine with me. I don't like birthday parties. Few things feel more horrifying to me than waiting out the thirty seconds it takes for a group of people to sing "Happy Birthday" to you in public.

It was easy to avoid making big b'day plans that year since I had a sinus infection, as did 99.9 percent of people in Manhattan in early December. My joints were unusually stiff and sore, which I attributed to being a fat girl who worked out. My energy tank was empty, no surprise considering my workload. On my résumé: I was writing a series pilot for VH1 with my friend Lizz. Our first professional collaboration had been a talk show/sitcom pilot for MTV, starring a studly male VJ who later became famous for making a gay porn video (one day we writers hung out in a conference room and watched him indifferently masturbate on TV). I was performing in a play at a SoHo theater. A story I'd written for *BUST* was about to be published in an anthology. I'd produced a small indie film called *flushed*, directed by my friend Carrie, who had recently moved out to L.A. The film had just been sold for distribution. I was also a freelancing for Lifetime Television's promo department; I awed myself with the number of hilarious promo lines I could write about 'round-the-clock *Golden Girls* episodes and movies starring Tiffani-Amber Thiessen. So, instead of one big bash, I booked lots of mini-events with my favorite people. Samantha, my best friend from college, gave me a big pink feather boa. My friend Marta, the other girl who could hold her own among our group of comedian guy friends, took me out to lunch. My brother, Josh, took me out to dinner. My parents had given me a beautiful winter coat when I'd been home in Detroit over Thanksgiving. My übercreative pals Bret and Tami, who I'd known since high school, sewed up a bag from scratch with a cartoon picture of me silk-screened onto it with the words THE WENDY SHANKER SHOW. They knew having my own TV show was the career path I dreamed about. Our other high school pal Marybeth stuffed the bag with a hot toddy kit (tea, honey, lemon, and a bottle of brandy) to help me get rid of my cold. Their gift was so original that I cried.

I also went out for a prepromised-no-singing birthday dinner
at a little downtown joint with my friend Emmy and her parents.
Emmy and I met in an improvisational comedy class and fell into
immediate girl crush mode. Her mom, Gerry, was a major player
in the TV industry who was developing a new television/Internet
channel for women called Oxygen. (Why "Oxygen"? Because you
need it. Because it's everywhere.) Over dessert, Gerry asked if I'd
be interested in writing a Web column (the term *blog* had yet to
be coined) that could one day translate into an on-air gig on her
channel-to-be. Would I? *Not much!* Are you kidding? I'd been so
depressed, wondering if all my efforts at writing, performing, and
producing would ever pay off, and here was a major opportunity!
I celebrated Gerry's potential offer by eating ice cream (Chubby
Hubby flavor; I certainly related to the "chubby" part), then got
mad at myself the minute I was done. The next day, I bought a
couple of size 22/24 skirts in case I'd have any start-up network
meetings to attend. I renewed my workout commitment for the
umpteenth time. Had to get my act together for the New Year.
I took a guy home after a Christmas party but couldn't really get
my hot hookup vibe going because I was busy thinking, Light in
my eye . . . fat . . . stubble scraping my face . . . fat . . . keep that
hand moving . . . fat . . . sigh . . . fat . . . and trying to elegantly
remove my control-top panty hose without killing the mood.
After he left, I flicked on the TV. *Men Don't Leave* was on, this
sad movie starring Jessica Lange as a mom who has to keep her
family together after the dad dies. The end makes me weep every
time, when the little boy looks up and asks his mother about his
late father: "Does he know I'm in the fourth grade?" I glanced at

my control tops balled in the corner of the couch. Yes. Men do leave.

I spent Christmas Eve with Emmy and her family, then Christmas Day with my friend Randy (whom I'd known since middle school) at our pal Joe's house in New Jersey. Joe worked at MTV and was a crazy Madonna fan like me. I was still exhausted from what felt like a never-frickin'-ending cold. Joe's mom cooked up a huge feast, and just when we thought we were finished, she brought out the *second* course. It's the Italian way! As a Jew, I always feel like Jane Goodall when I participate in a non-Jewish family's event. But I love being a part of the festivities. Christmas is great. It bites Hanukkah's ass.

My resolution for 1999 was simple: Be a phenomenal woman, per Maya Angelou's urging. But I wasn't starting out on a phenomenal foot. My damn sinus infection was entrenched. I'd churned through an array of antibiotics that my primary doctor had prescribed. The pain in my face was wearing me down, so I hunted down an ear/nose/throat (ENT) specialist. It was the week between Christmas and New Year's, which is a terrible time to sign up with a new doctor. Any medic worth his or her salt hightails it to Kauai or Cozumel and only newbies or second-tier clinicians lurk around New York during the holidays.

The ENT I met vibed the low energy of an office drone killing time to reach his twenty-five-year mark so he could receive a low-end Rolex and escape into retirement. His office reminded me of a garage that had been converted from an off-to-college son's bedroom into dad's "office." The doctor poked around inside my nose and throat and surmised, "You need a CT scan. I see some errant tissue in the airway." In other words, something was jammed in my sinuses, like when my brother was little and shoved a dime up his nose. My dad had to get up in there with a pair of pliers and yank the coin out.

A couple of days later, while waiting at a radiology office to get the CT scan that would hopefully explain my eternal sinus infection, I impatiently flipped through women's magazines from 1997 with Kim Basinger and Minnie Driver on the covers. One was a special we-don't-really-mean-it-but-we'll-pretend-this-month-we'll-celebrate-it "Body Issue." Flip. Flip. Flip. I had to get back to work. The receptionist assured me I'd be seen momentarily, and added, "What a beautiful round face you have!" I'm sorry, a beautiful round face? Now there's a fresh spin on the passive-aggressive "What a pretty face!" comment. I instantly deflated. I was so far from phenomenal. I had a "phenomenal" phobia. The truth is, it didn't matter what great idea I conceived or what job I landed. I was too fat. *Fat.* As I lay frozen in the giant CT tunnel, I realized I had to turn my life around. Meridia, the appetite suppressant I was taking, wasn't helping at all. I'd heard about an adult fat farm in North Carolina at Duke University. People went there as a last-ditch effort and supposedly lost a lot of weight, a final stop on the permanent road to weight loss. I needed to go hard-core. I had no energy, no spirit. I was sick of feeling sick. My spunky cousin Alex in Michigan had lost her leg and died from cancer at only seventeen; I had no excuse for holding back. I'd never be successful or happy if I wasn't thin and beautiful. I would call Duke in the morning.

JANUARY 1999

The CT scan revealed a mystery chunk in my sinuses: "Diffuse soft tissue fullness involving the nasal septum particularly anteriorly at the level of the cartilaginous septum . . . the possibility of granulomatous disease is raised," according to the radiology report (I'll stick with "mystery chunk"; it's much more fun). I upgraded to a more experienced surgical ENT, Dr. Wilson, for a follow-up biopsy. Biopsy, schmiopsy. No biggie. Here's how much I wasn't scared: I went to the procedure by myself. Took the M72 bus across Central Park to Lenox Hill Hospital. While I was sedated, the surgeon scooped out a chunk of the chunk, then packed my nose full of gauze and bandaged it, leaving me with the black-eyed and tissue-stuffed appearance of all the girls in high school who'd had their noses done. He jammed my nose so full of gauze and ointment that it stretched as wide as my mouth. I didn't look pretty or feel comfortable, but I could deal. I was lucky enough to have the all-day postsurgical services of my friend Nurse Tami. Bret and Marybeth got me a little gift to cheer me up. Emmy stopped by with flowers. Samantha sent some, too. Tami intercepted a zillion concerned phone calls while I slept off the anesthesia. I couldn't imagine what I'd done to be on the receiving end of so much attention and love.

I didn't bother to go back to the doc for a postsurgical follow-up as directed; instead I pulled all the packing out myself. I'm the kind of person who would not only remove her own stitches, but collect them in a scrapbook. I would've kept the dime from my brother's nose and framed it. It's a little *Silence of the Lambs* creepy. But I couldn't see any reason not to pull advanced-caliber Kleenex out of my nose.

I was still black and blue, but examining myself in the mirror while degauzing, I could already see I was healing. When Dr. Wilson prepped me for the biopsy, he'd told me, "Don't worry. It's not cancer." Oh—was I supposed to be thinking it was cancer? My priority was finding a time to zip out of New York and hit up that weight rehab program at Duke.

Back to other people's business, as celebrity gossip data came in handy on most of my writing gigs. Ben Affleck broke up with Gwyneth Paltrow, then started doing Pilates and juice fasts. Gwyneth was thrilled with a Fifty-seventh Street beauty salon, The J Sisters, which specialized in extremely bare bikini waxes. I imagined Gwyneth holding up a palm in "girlfriend, please" position and raving to a pal: "You should *see* my vagina." To kick off the New Year, Rosie O'Donnell started a "Chub Club" on her daytime talk show. I was certainly eligible to join, but I didn't want to belong to a club with that name even if they'd have me (they would—I was clocking in around 241). Ro was still friends with Mo (Madonna), and she and O(prah) got superfriendly after they bonded on O's show. In a new take on self-improvement, Oprah suggested writing in "gratitude journals" and remembering our spirit. Her mantra: "Oh God, my heart is open to you. Come sit in my heart." I could remember that one.

My friend Mark worked in the press office at the White House and tipped me off that a massive news story was about to break. He was right. President Clinton got dressed down for getting a BJ from an intern in the Oval Office. As a curvy Jewess with brown hair, I was often confused with that naughty intern. Comedy producers asked me if I could dress up as Monica Lewinsky at upcoming showcases. I went to Bloomingdale's and stuffed myself into a lavender two-piece Tahari suit that looked *sooo* Monica. I'd return it after the audition. Disturbingly, my joints were so sore that I could barely get off the bus to try out at those auditions. The subway was no longer an option for me; there was no way I could get up and down the stairs in this much pain. If I didn't get the part, fine, I'd go to Duke. I'd lose weight, so no one would ever mistake me for Monica again.

I didn't get the part. I started researching airfares to North Carolina.

D<small>r.</small> Wilson delivered my official diagnosis in an emerald-green-carpeted room. I squirmed around in a leather chair, trying to find a position that would soothe my joints. The doctor wore a green tie that matched the carpet. He was a tall, lean, older man who still had all his hair. Nicely done. He smiled and paused. "Well, Miss Shanker, your biopsy shows 'inflamed mucosa, largely necrotic with multinucleated giant cells of Langhans type, suggestive of a disease called Wegener's granulomatosis.'"

"Wegenah what?" I repeated. I don't know what I was expecting to hear, but it wasn't whatever that guy just said.

"It's a fairly rare autoimmune disease. To tell you the truth, I don't know much about it. But I know a rheumatologist in the city who does—here's his contact information." He jotted down a name and number on his prescription pad and pushed it toward me: Howard Baker. Wilson concluded, "Go see him and he'll tell you what to do. I just have one piece of advice: Do *not* start looking this up on the Internet."

I could not get home fast enough to go online. All I knew was that I had some disease that started with a *W* and that I'd probably need to find a Jew to fix it. I used my dial-up modem to connect to the Internet, which I still really didn't know how to use. It was 1999, people. I was sending e-mails, but I'd rarely surfed into the vast sea of information of things that started with "w-w-w." This was an era when the Dancing Baby on *Ally McBeal* seemed like a triumph of technology. I slowly typed in the name of the disease that the doc had spelled out for me in his office: "W-E-G-E-N-E-R-S." Sounded German. Figures the Nazis would be behind this whole thing.*

---

* Actually, the Nazis *were* behind this whole thing! "In 2000, Dr. Eric Matteson, a rheumatologist at the Mayo Clinic, and Dr. Alexander Woywodt, a kidney specialist now living in England, set out to write a column celebrating Wegener for *The Lancet*, the British medical journal. They uncovered a Nazi past that Wegener had kept secret after World War II. Unlike doctors who joined the Nazi Party to be allowed to practice, Wegener joined the movement in 1932, before Hitler took power.

The Cleveland Clinic website described the illness this way: "Wegener's granulomatosis is an extremely rare disease of uncertain cause. It is characterized by an inflammation in a variety of tissues, including blood vessels (vasculitis). Inflammation damages vital organs of the body by restricting blood flow to those organs. Although vasculitis can damage any organ system, Wegener's granulomatosis primarily affects the respiratory tract (sinus, nose, trachea, lungs) and the kidneys." It could also affect the joints as rheumatoid arthritis does, which explained the agony I'd been feeling. Here I'd been thinking it was osteoarthritis pain that I deserved for being fat and putting undue pressure on joints. Always easy to blame myself.

A few newspaper articles had been scanned and posted online on patient community sites. I read about missing limbs and chemotherapy treatments. I noted terms like *incurable*, *tracheotomy*, and *life expectancy*. Minimal research revealed that I'd been lucky to get a diagnosis at all, let alone within a few months of onset of my initial symptoms. Most people found out they had Wegener's the hard way: in other words, dying in a gurney in the hallway of some hospital. There was no specific profile for a Wegener's patient; 97 percent of the people who had it were Caucasian, evenly spread among women and men. Eighty-five

He rose to a relatively high military rank and spent some of the war in a medical office three blocks from the Jewish ghetto in Lodz, Poland. Sketchy records suggest that he might have participated in experiments on concentration camp inmates." Barnaby J. Feder, "A Nazi Past Casts a Pall on Name of a Disease," *New York Times*, January 22, 2008.

percent were above age nineteen, with a median age of forty-one. They lived in no particular part of the country. Wegener's wasn't contagious and wasn't necessarily caused by anything genetic. Researchers thought it could possibly be triggered by a virus that some bodies couldn't fend off, or toxins in the environment. Hmm, I did have that weird mono my final semester of college. Maybe that had been the start of the Wegener's? Could it be bad tuna? Toxic paint? Why, of all things, this? Apparently, there was only one proven way to treat this vascular autoimmune disease: steroids + chemo.

I shared this information with my intimate circle of friends and family, who shot into immediate help mode. Tami talked to friends at the hospital where she worked. My aunt Nancy consulted colleagues in Atlanta and North Carolina from her RN days. In Detroit, my distressed dad and stepmom, Mickey and Myrna, reached out to their network in Michigan's Jewish community. Treatment options began rolling in. Emotionally and physically drained, sore from my aching joints, I was angry that Dr. Wilson didn't have more information for me, and was frustrated to be thrust into potential life limbo. How long was I was going to have to pull out of my daily routine to treat this problem . . . six or seven *months*? What would I do for money? What about all of my potential TV show ideas and phenomenal woman career plans? And who on earth would want to date a twenty-seven-year-old sick chick? Plus I'd already gone ahead and made that reservation at the Duke Diet & Fitness Center. I was hunting for freelance TV jobs and hoping the Oxygen thing might work out. Now I had to worry about stuff like remedies and remissions? I felt stagnant and loserish, lame and scared. I didn't know how to be a good soldier quite yet.

I envisioned two possible futures for myself (so Gwyneth *Sliding Doors*). The first: I would be one of the easy, "limited" cases the literature talked about. I'd have sinus problems or whatever, but Wegener's would never affect my kidneys. I'd take this prednisone steroid thing and probably a chemo drug called Cytoxan. It would suck, I'd get fatter (at least I'd have a decent excuse), then I'd get over it and go into remission, forever. The title of this story? "So, Not the Greatest Thing." The End.

The alternative: There was already something wrong with my lungs. My nose would collapse (it was already looking a little mushy and shifting to the left). I could handle fat and pretty, but now I would be fat and ugly—unbearable. I'd be unable to drop the steroid weight. I'd develop osteoporosis and cataracts. I'd never get my period again and I wouldn't be able to have kids. That made me cry. I could still live a long time, but my lonely, older years would be filled with pain and discomfort.

You'd think that the fear of that second path would inspire me to work out more, sleep right, eat kale and radishes and all that shit. Nah. I wasn't going to turn into one of those annoying people who schlepped yoga mats around SoHo in those little mesh bags. "Check me out, I do *yoga*." No, thanks. Mostly I felt chagrined to have my life interrupted. I had stuff to do: meetings with Oxygen; working with the media team at V-Day, Eve Ensler's effort to end violence against women and girls; consulting with a plus-size women's magazine called *Mode*; writing a Jewish teens' website advice column ("Tell Aviv!"); participating in a feminist reading at this cool bar in the East Village—livin' the dream, baby! But . . . sometimes I felt short of breath. Was that because I had a tumor in my lungs? Or was it my imagination? Was the pain shooting up my leg from rheumatoid arthritis, or too many hours sauntering around on John Fleuvog platform boots?

This wasn't the first time illness had deeply affected my life. As I mentioned, my mom (or as my aunt Nancy calls her, my "bio-mom") died when I was ten years old. My brother was only eight. We weren't prepared; she'd been diagnosed with leukemia a year and a half earlier when she'd gone to the doctor for her annual ob-gyn checkup, and got weird results back on her Pap smear. Doctors told my parents she had only three to five years (talk about Death Math), but she felt fine. She and my father had opted to keep her diagnosis a secret. They figured they'd wait until she was so sick it was obvious, and then they'd confess. It didn't play out that way. One day she got the flu, the next day she went into the hospital, and the following night my dad came home and told me that she had died. Along with the shock of losing a woman who we thought was a healthy thirty-five-year-old, her death held an element of martyrdom. She had spared her parents, her children, and her friends the pain and worry that came with knowing she was sick. She had selflessly protected us. But by keeping her illness a secret, she had also taken away our opportunity to let her go.

Aunts and neighbors tried to comfort me by explaining that God needed Mommy, so He had to take her "away." "Away" was somewhere vaguely up and over, as if she'd booked a trip to a remote island near Hawaii that couldn't be reached by phone. If we could find her somewhere over the rainbow, maybe there was a chance that she could come back home. I was bewildered. According to my estimates, God had five billion people to choose from. He'd needed my mother to fulfill some particular role for Him that no one else—say, someone who was not a mother of two small children—could play? My mom was a consummate hostess, a vibrant conversationalist, an organized and engaged woman who loved being a parent. But unless God needed her to make a three-tiered Jell-O mold (lemon with pineapple, Cool Whip, and blackberry with blackberries, which sounds gross but is crazy delicious), or carpool to Miss Barbara's Dance Centre on Thursdays, I couldn't figure out why she was the only girl for the gig.

Maybe Death was like the draft, and even flat feet or moving to Canada wouldn't get her out of duty. Maybe she'd fought God valiantly, explaining that she had responsibilities to attend to in real life, like shopping for my back-to-school clothes and raising money for the Pine Lake Elementary book fair. But since God was more powerful, more even than Mommy or Daddy, she had to go.

Or maybe . . . what if the draft was voluntary, and Mommy had chosen God over us? She was simply so selfless that she gave herself up to help someone who needed her way more than we did. She must have been sure we were strong enough to go on without her. No, it was unthinkable that she hadn't put up a fight, or worse, that the whole "away" thing wasn't true. If all this God stuff was made up, then she was just dead. A mammal whose cells had backfired and mutated her out of existence. There had to be a sensible reason for her death that was simply beyond my ten-year-old comprehension level. Nothing I knew could justify something so unexplainably bad happening.

Her loss gave me an E-ZPass on emotional suffering, and nothing could really hurt me after that. My pain scale had been instantly and radically altered. I couldn't point to the chart and give it a number. Normal preteen stuff still bugged me: memorizing presidents, getting picked last for gym, hoping that Kiki McGraw would invite me to her birthday sleepover. But I quickly became immune to the interior aches of adolescence, the kind my friends had: boys not liking them back, parents splitting up, dads losing jobs, moms gaining weight. At least they had their moms.

I still believe that despite all of the therapy, communication, and openness that have become common in the last twenty-five years, and the luck we had in my dad marrying Myrn, my family was doomed to screw this one up. No one does death right, especially "out of the natural order of things" death. We were a perfect Mommy-Daddy-little-girl-little-boy-little-dog family living in a nice suburb in the Midwest in 1982. *Ordinary People* had just won an Oscar. This was before Oprah, before Self-Help had its own section in the bookstore, before you could click for daily Deepak Chopra updates online. The cultural vibe was repress, repress, confront, and then repress some more. My mom had been angry with me when she found her copy of *Love Story* in my nightstand. (Not as furious as when she found a tampon in my jewelry box—I had no clue what the thing was, but I found it under the sink in Sherri Lavine's guest bathroom, and kept it as evidence . . . just in case.) I thought my mom was mad at me because there was a sex scene in the book. Now I know it was because *Love Story* was her story. She was the Jewish Ali MacGraw, a brilliant beauty secretly dying of leukemia. My dad was the Jewish Ryan O'Neal, hiding his pain, too in love to let her go.

As a kid, it didn't occur to me to be angry with my parents. No one owed me an apology (after all, love means never having to say you're sorry) for my mom hiding such a major secret, then dying. No forgiving necessary. There was no guidebook to tell us what to do, no rules like for how to play four-square or sell Girl Scout cookies. So I planted a smile on my face and kept on going. I didn't know I had options (e.g., public tantrums, drinking beer with the bad kids in the parking lot of the 7-Eleven, making Lolita eyes at a family friend). I liked being good. My mother had taken pride in my excellent grades and nice manners. I still wanted her to love me. So I did what I would have done if she were still there: put barrettes in my hair, walked out of the house, and started the sixth grade.

Now I was almost at the age she was when she died, and I was sick, too. The issue of "choice" about the situation came up again. Did something in me choose to be sick? Friends who did stuff like yoga and Reiki thought there was a connection between physical health and emotional health: "If your body is sick, maybe your heart is, too." Ergo, if I could fix my heart, I could fix my health. But that didn't ring true for me. I'd already gone to therapy. I'd journaled, I'd taken Method acting classes, I did some self-searching. I talked and cried and grieved as much as I knew how. I thought my energy was clean, but I got sick anyway. What did I have to do now, up the ante and explore past lives, karmic destiny, and astrological charts to see if I missed a spot somewhere? Wasn't my style. Fix what's broken and get on with it; that was my MO. What mystical healers would call "pods of sadness" or "living in the fourth chakra of grief," I called lung tumors. I understood the symbolism of disease: a broken heart, sick to your stomach, a pain in the ass. But I didn't believe that emotions could literally cause illness. So the solution seemed clear: Prescribe me the pill, give me the shot, or cut out the bad parts and move on.

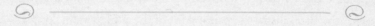

## FEBRUARY 1999

Happy Valentine's Day 1999, because everyone in the entire universe is erotically loved and adored—except for me! Mick and Myrn flew in from Detroit for a visit. Myrn roasted up a turkey. Mick gave me a Valentine's Barbie doll. How cute is that? He watched this new HBO mob drama called *The Sopranos* while I listened to *The Miseducation of Lauryn Hill* nonstop.

A fat packet arrived in my mailbox from the Wegener's Granulomatosis Support Group headquarters in Kansas City, Missouri; I'd sent away for it through the mail, as there was no website. Clearly the support group was a small-time operation; the materials included a welcome note and a pile of much-photocopied articles about people who had been diagnosed with Wegener's and the treatment protocols they'd followed. HOLDING DEATH AT BAY was a headline from one patient profile in a local paper. ILLNESS IMPRISONS LOCAL MAN, read another. They'd included cartoons, poems, and inspirational quotes, and articles like "When Sorrows Call: Strategies for Survival" and "Taming the Medical Debt Monster."

An opening letter written by Marilyn Sampson, the support group's founder, read: "We are not some big fancy support group. We are just people caring for people and we want to help you in any way we can. . . . A very serious disease has struck, and we will be here to give you all of the support we can through this difficult time. We know the feeling of isolation and fear of the unknown with you or someone in your family having Wegener's. This is normal when dealing with a rare disease like we have. Know that long-term remission can be obtained; there is hope. You must believe this!" A lovely letter, but I didn't have any "isolation" or "fear of the unknown" until after I read it. What unmoored me was a postscript that said: "Marilyn Sampson, R.N., passed away October 7, 1997 after a long bout with cancer (not caused by Wegener's)." Terribly sad news . . . but oh my God, were they absolutely sure that she died from cancer and not Wegener's?

One of the articles clipped from a 1986 issue of *People* was about a girl my age who had been diagnosed with Wegener's when she was in high school. "From the time she was 12," it read, "Michele's life has been a litany of pain and a catalog of hospitals. A rare cancer-like disease that attacks cartilage had disfigured her by destroying her sinuses, windpipe and eventually her nose. She would have to attend the sorority rush party with an artificial nose held to her face by magnets implanted in her skull. . . ."

She *attended* the *sorority rush party*!? I would have driven myself off a cliff.

It got better.

"For a while Michele made do with a Band-Aid over her facial hole. Five months later [the surgeon] tried a new technique, implanting a stainless-steel pin, about as thick as cardboard, with a rare-earth magnet containing the metallic element cobalt, to which an artificial nose could be held. He also reconstructed Michele's voice box, reaming out scar tissue 'as hard as cement' and replacing it with a plastic tube wrapped with skin graft."

You're telling me . . . Michele's nose had literally fallen off her face, Michael Jackson–style? Then clever surgeons had implanted a magnet in her skull so she could hook different noses on her face, depending on her mood, like day-of-the-week underpants? Wouldn't it be a safer bet to affix the nose with Krazy Glue, like the guy in the commercial wearing the helmet and hanging off the underside of a girder? This girl had balls. She'd hooked on an aquiline honker, wheeled herself to rush, and pledged a sorority! Oy, Michele!

I was horrified, but I wasn't scared. Puh-leeze. I certainly wasn't going to end up a wheelchair-riding, dialysis-getting, nose-magnet-wearing Wegener's sufferer. Right? But . . . what if I did? I didn't have the deep-seated confidence of someone like Michele, who would fight back and triumph over the odds just to be a part of an Alpha Beta Omega Four-Way Greek Week kegger. I wasn't a warrior; I was a wuss. When I watch disaster movies, I always pray that if I were in that situation—crashed on a desert island, adrift at sea, or stranded with a team of soccer players in the Andes—my comrades would put me out of my misery and eat me first.

I surmised those stories in the Wegener's packet had to be extreme cases, rare scenarios. Wegener's was a chronic sinus issue. It wasn't a death sentence like . . . cancer. Or leukemia. I had to be rational. Clearly there was something wrong with my body that was going to give me hella trouble. I just had to fix it. It was like being fat. I'd been fighting my weight since puberty, so it wasn't like I'd ever had a positive mind/body connection; it wasn't gonna start now. My body always felt like a car engine to me. I had to take decent care of it for it to work well. If something was broken, it could be repaired. If I didn't like the way it looked (and I never did) I could get a new paint job. I was basically a car with a brain, a fat Jewish version of Kitt on *Knight Rider*. Okay. I could handle this. I clearly had an annoying and potentially frustrating journey ahead of me, but I'd just have to keep things stable, then find a Hasselhoffian way to turn this baby around and drive off into the horizon.

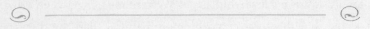

MARCH 1999

Finally, my appointment with Dr. Howard Baker, a highly lauded rheumatologist in New York medical circles. I still wasn't exactly sure what arena of medicine rheumatology covered; I recalled reading a lot of nineteenth-century novels in college where characters had "rheumy eyes" or "rheumatic fever" or the mystifying catchall "rheumatism." I deduced that a rheumatologist specialized in goo. I was close. Doctors generally don't use the term *goo*, but rheumatology is a study of connective tissues and joints. Other patients went to rheumatologists to treat lupus, rheumatoid arthritis, multiple sclerosis, and other rare minidiseases I'd never heard of.

This older, warmer doctor gave me the overview: I had "limited" Wegener's, meaning the disease hadn't affected my kidneys. He ordered a CT scan of my chest and abdomen to be sure my other organs were okay. We did a bone-density scan to set a baseline. Since Wegener's could also affect the eyes, he suggested I schedule an ophthalmological exam. Baker confirmed that Wegener's wasn't curable but was treatable, with potentially long remissions between flares. No need for scary Cytoxan yet; the first line of defense was a sulfa drug called Bactrim. Sulfa, as in sulfur. It's a classic old-school pharmaceutical that basically burns away the bad stuff. It only took two days for me to develop a head-to-toe rash that made me look like a lobster crossed with a Seurat painting. Wow, my first known allergy! I look back on this burn fondly. It was my first whiplash of Western medicine, when I suspected that the cures could be more harmful than the diseases themselves.

I cut off the Bactrim and shifted to the next drug on Baker's combat list: methotrexate (MTX), a low-grade chemotherapeutic drug (sometimes used to induce abortions); and prednisone, a corticosteroid meant to control the inflammation in my joints that was causing my arthritis pain. Vascular diseases create inflammation in the blood vessels, which cuts off blood to the organs, leading to organ damage. As an extra-special added gift, Wegener's forges a kind of inflammatory tissue in blood vessels called granulomas, which destroy normal tissue. Why? Because the immune system thinks it's attacking an outsider. Unfortunately, it's just attacking you. "Oops, got the wrong message. Sorry." Corticosteroids simulate the hormone cortisol, which is naturally produced by the adrenal gland, and thus slows down the body's immune system so it just might stop damaging itself. The steroid thing was massively confusing: I wasn't a bodybuilder or a professional baseball player, so why did I need steroids to enhance my performance? Turns out there's a difference between prednisone, the anti-inflammatory drug that I'd be taking, and the human growth hormones and steroids that half the players in Major League Baseball take (or don't take; whatever, guys).

On methotrexate and prednisone, I still had shooting pains in my right knee, hip, and shoulder. I started feeling nauseous. My skin became very fragile. I wasn't going to town Brazilian bikini– style, J Sister-ing it up à la Gwyneth, but Olga at Salon Selina nearly ripped my forehead off when I went for an eyebrow wax. The rest of my body started looking . . . furry. My nose discharged all sorts of weird gunk. My eyes were dry and itchy; I was parched and thirsty. I still had the remnants of my Bactrim rash all over my torso. My vagina was a tingle fest (not in a good way) and my head killed. Blood tests revealed that my liver enzymes were elevated—I didn't know what that signified, but I knew it wasn't good. But again, not cancer. Actually, I felt guilty that the diagnosis wasn't worse, the kind of thing that could take me down before I hit thirty-five. Shh, don't tell God.

My urine test came back abnormal—and it took a week to get the results. So frustrating. What if the Wegener's bypassed my lungs and skipped straight to my kidneys? Was that even possible? Dr. Baker put me on a higher dose of methotrexate, just in case. Then my septum officially perforated. I saw a picture of it on a video screen at the ENT's office. They said there wasn't much more I could do than irrigate my sinuses with a "nasal douche," a tool in need of a much cooler name. I could just imagine my nightly routine: "Sorry, sweetheart, I'll come to bed in a second— first I have to *nasal douche*." On the cool side, I could stick a Q-tip through my septum. Don't ask me how I figured that out. You don't want to know.

Concerned friends and family members continued to weigh in with the Best Guys they knew and the Best Places I should go and the Best Drugs from articles they'd read. Notes and paperwork related to autoimmune research started to pile up on my desk. Acquaintances who embraced alternative and complementary healing suggested their own treatment opinions ("Raw food!" "Echinacea!" "Hypnosis!"). I was advised to change my diet, beauty, and hygiene products and wardrobe, or just plain up and move to a prairie somewhere. Myrn recalled a cold I had in 1998 when I went to Prague with Carrie to promote *flushed*, and wondered if that could have been the root of it (Nazis strike again!). I got a second (third, fourth) opinion from another well-regarded rheumatologist, every year listed as one of "New York's Best," who assured me that I never would have contracted Wegener's granulomatosis if I weren't so fat. Lovely guy. He warned me, "Prednisone won't make you gain weight. It's your appetite that does it." His admonition only served to reinforce my sense of helplessness.

I quickly had to develop a filter on the ambient input and figure out a diplomatic way to tell people I loved to shut the F up. I understand the instinct to want to help fix people when something is broken. I long to help sick friends get healthier, or sad friends get happier. But everyone I spoke to was convinced she was an expert. I know the feeling; you click on some link that catches your attention on the AOL home page and think, "Why didn't my doctor tell me about . . . uh, cactus juice cocktails? Is he dumb? Is he out of the loop? Does he even have e-mail?" But having been diagnosed with a rare, incurable disease, I chose to believe that doctors were the experts. They were the brains that graduated from medical school. Not me, not my doorman, not my friend-of-a-friend. If my physicians chose to ignore a symptom or prescribe a particular drug, I was going to follow their directions, despite my own misgivings or other people's "been there, done that" directives. Every time I met an "expert," whether it was for weight loss, therapy, or now this Wegener's stuff, I secretly hoped that he or she was the One who would instantly know the right answer and give me the quick fix. If only I could find the right expert, I could be thin/happy/healthy. Since I'd never managed to fix myself, it never occurred to me that *I* might be the expert.

D r. Baker was transitioning out of his practice and handing off new patients to his accomplished partner, Dr. Daniel Turner. I liked Turner right off the bat. He was tall and handsome and completely unpretentious, with a Woody Allen–ish New York accent. He sat on the examining table as we talked. I liked that. Most doctors conferred with me across an expanse of desk. Or else I'd be on the examining table while he or she stood in front of me, a situation that lent the doc authority and left me vulnerable. By sitting on the exam table, it was like Turner was putting himself in my shoes. We discussed the intensity and treatment risks of different drug regimens, and how they would affect other issues like bone density. I soon became familiar with diagnostic tools like ANCA (an antibody test used to determine potential for active Wegener's) and sedimentation rate (which could indicate an infection in my system). I spent a thousand uninsured dollars to pay a visit to a fertility specialist. If I would one day have to do chemotherapy, I wanted to keep my procreation options open. The fertility specialist breezily told me, "Don't bother freezing your eggs if you don't have anyone to fertilize them." Again, not necessarily a diplomatic doc. Plus, hell-o? At that time, a major decision for me was whether to get chips with my sandwich in the MTV/Viacom cafeteria. I hadn't exactly picked out my Future Fertilizer.

Even while I was on prednisone and methotrexate, nasty sinusitis continued to gain ground. Turner sent me to an ENT he often worked with named Barry Allen, the otolaryngological

Butch Cassidy to his rheumatological Sundance Kid. Allen belonged to a large otolaryngology practice across the street from St. Luke's–Roosevelt Hospital. Dr. Allen cared for most of the known Wegener's patients in the tristate area. Even other doctors in his ENT practice were unfamiliar with the disease. "I'm just a plumber," Allen humbly referred to himself. "I fix the pipes." He deferred to Dr. Turner to deal with the artistry of diagnosis and medication.

Every time I went to see Dr. Allen, I studied the people in the waiting room and wondered what was wrong with their ears, noses, and throats. Bad case of laryngitis got ya down? Poor baby. Stuck a Q-tip too far into your eardrum? That's a shame. I learned to carry lots of reading materials with me to doctors' waiting rooms, as cell phones were verboten and the only literature I could find in the lobby were old issues of *Car & Driver* and *American Way*, the in-flight magazine for American Airlines. Sometimes in Allen's waiting room I'd spot an elderly man jealously eyeballing my *New York Post*, so I'd nonchalantly leave it on the chair as if I'd just picked it up there in the first place. It was my way of showing solidarity with other people who were physically screwed above the neck.

This ENT's suite looked like a dentist's office: a big execution-style chair in the middle and a cabinet off to the side where pointy and painful-looking tools waited to get popped into my upper orifices. Each office featured posters of sinus and inner-ear diagrams on the wall. My favorite was the one with the progressive photos of disintegrating inner ears—everything looks like Bubble Yum at first, but then devolves into green oyster meat.

The good news about having a doctor poke around in your ears and nose and down your throat is that there aren't a lot of nerve endings. The bad news is, there are *some*. Dr. Allen would stuff a hose into my ear canal to suck fluid out of it. Head-spin inducing, and not very fun. My only consolation was begging him to attach the video monitor extension to the nasal probe so I could see the cavities of my nose and get a close-up view of my vocal cords. FYI, everything inside the body pretty much looks like a vagina.

"The inflammation has improved in here," he'd say, poking into my nose with a nasal speculum. (Really, I never thought I'd have to deal with more than one kind of speculum in my life.) I was always impressed that Allen could distinguish the changes in my ethmoid sinus from appointment to appointment. I once asked a therapist how she was able to remember the names of family members, friends, and coworkers whom I would rant about during our appointments. She said, "Don't you remember all the names of the family members and coworkers that your friends have? You remember details about people that you care about." With Allen, it was like my sinus cavities were my bloody, discharging, necrotizing little friends, and each one had a special place in his heart. Having found my experts, I religiously went to my appointments, took my medications, and waited for a more awful and life-threatening disease to come along.

# 2

## Borderline

MAY 1999

That spring, Brad Pitt met Jennifer Aniston, and Gwyneth got an Oscar as a consolation prize. I did improv comedy shows, worked on my one-woman show, wrote articles about pop culture for women's magazines, and started building Web concepts for Oxygen, where I'd landed a dreamy development gig. The network had purchased a women's entertainment website that they wanted me to overhaul and supervise. With so much work to do, I had to put off my trip to Duke. But in welcome news, Turner had given me an optimistic report. My ANCA level, the blood test that searched for white blood cell antibodies, had dropped. He said, "We can even start thinking about remission."

In that spirit I went to my first Wegener's support group meeting, held in a conference room at Allen's office. A committee member had purchased big two-liter bottles of generic soda pop and soft little plastic cups. About thirty generic people sat around in a circle. Their faces reflected Wegener's features and attitudes:

soft, flat and exhausted. Cosmetically, I was a hot mess. Not just my face—due to prednisone, from head to toe I looked like the Pillsbury Dough Girl. Turner and Allen spoke for a few minutes; then the audience asked questions to which I already knew the answers. On my way out, Allen patted me on the shoulder and assured me, "Don't worry, you'll get off prednisone and your clothes will fit you again." I was like, Honey. What do you think? This isn't swelling from steroids. This is me. Fat and zitty, with huge rips across my stomach—big purple stretch marks. Plus, in a rare aberration, I didn't like the haircut Dorothy had given me. I'd made the mistake of saying, "Why don't we try something new?" It was way too short, and kind of feathered in the front. I couldn't look more wrong at the moment. It was like every force had turned against me when it was so obvious that beauty was the key to work, love, everything. So why had I resisted for so long, fought so hard to stay fat? Why was I so lazy, such a sucker to my appetite? Why hadn't I stuck to diets, gotten surgery, did whatever it was that made entertainment execs want to hire you, audiences laugh at you, and guys pick you up in bars? The night before, when I sat down with friends at dinner in a Theater District restaurant, the hostess crouched down and asked me, "Would you be more comfortable switching to a chair without arms?" Brightly, I chirped, "No, thank you"—but burned with humiliation in front of my friends. So I put in a call to the doctor's office to explore my umpteenth round of doctor-supervised Optifast protein starvation shakes. Surely I'd lose major poundage on only five hundred calories a day. I debated joining Overeater's Anonymous just to cover my (big fat) ass.

The following week Oxygen upped my job ante: Basically, they wanted me to do anything and everything, in every capacity. Write for TV shows and on the website. Produce. Develop programming with any team that needed me—production, promos, marketing. Still, no on-air time guaranteed. Effective Monday. I'd be on staff, for the first time ever, getting health benefits, a 401(k), the whole deal. No stock options, which were major currency in the new Internet job era—yet. A solid chunk of change in terms of salary—probably more than most of my friends earned. I had to come up with a job title: Renaissance Woman? Converger? Converged Thinker? Multitasker? Gerry had a suggestion: "Your title should be . . . 'Voice.' You're the voice of the network."

A part of me wasn't perfectly thrilled about the job offer. Fear of success? Nah. Maybe I'd been waiting too long for a dream job to come along. Maybe the steroids were messing with my logic. Maybe I was exhausted. Maybe I didn't know if I could handle it. . . . Oh please, I could definitely handle it. I was worried about losing my flexibility and freedom. Would I still have time to perform sets at clubs at night? Write my own one-woman shows? Maybe I'd been infused with freelance-style productivity for so long that I was afraid to plug in to a full-time gig. Plus I still had to sneak out to all those doctor's appointments. Only Gerry knew I was sick. I was trying to keep the Wegener's on the DL from my new coworkers. No one wants to work with a woman who may not be dependable enough to hold up her end of the gig.

Maybe structure would be good for me, and not only as a distraction from my health drama. I'd gotten so out of touch with my potential, my spark—that singular vibe that draws people to you. I'd been faking it over my negative (*fat fat fat*) interior monologue every second of every day for years. I wondered if this job could help me get my shit together. I'd figure out what my goals were, then get out there and achieve them. Some self-control might be a good start. I'd actually eaten almost perfectly that day. No crap, no binges. That was an improvement. Work kept me too busy to eat. At the end of our meeting about the job offer, my new almost-boss reached around and hugged me—and pulled back a forearm full of perspiration. I was always so hot and sweaty. It was so embarrassing. Maybe if I lost weight, I'd be cooler in more ways than one.

I met Sam for dinner, then went to see our friends Jason and Randy Sklar perform stand-up at a downtown comedy club. As I watched them, I wondered, Shouldn't I be doing stand-up, too? Did taking this office job mean I was giving up on a creative dream? No, I was on a different road. I had to stay confident in my choices. As I left the club, I spotted my Christmas party fling and gave him a wave. He ran the other way. Boys. So *stoopid*.

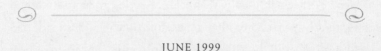

## JUNE 1999

joined my new colleagues at an upstate, upstart company retreat. I packed the biggest clothes I owned (three big, frumpy dresses) and all my medications. We were staying in a college dorm, but luckily I had a single, so no one would catch me with my stash. At a breakout session, we played a game called Enemy/ Protector. Without speaking to anyone, you had to select one person in the room to be your Enemy, and one to be your Protector. Then you had to physically keep your Protector between you and your Enemy at all times, which forced everyone to run around the room like electrons gone wild. I was running around like crazy, laughing—hard to do when I was that overheated and exhausted—before I realized that about a dozen people were running behind me. They had all picked me to be their Protector. Because of my girth? My personality? Both? I felt honored, then drained. Working this hard and feeling this crappy, it was going to get increasingly more challenging for me to take care of everyone else.

JULY 1999

Post-retreat, I had a follow-up appointment with Dr. Allen. Again he examined the inside of my nose with a scope. "Well, I see that perforation in your septum . . . and increased 'saddlenose deformity' as well." That meant a flattening across the bridge of my schnoz, called so because it looked like a saddle. Boxers had it from getting punched in the face, as did cokeheads who blew out their septums on nose candy.

"Is there anything I can do about it?" I asked.

"There are surgical procedures to repair it, but long-term success rates are low with Wegener's patients, whose bodies often reject implants. So we can't use plastic. We'd have to use bone from your hip or rib. It's okay. If it stays like this, no one will even notice."

Hello—Did the docs who'd done my biopsy just scoop out a hunk of my nose without considering I might need that hunk in the future? Allen also noted signs of chronic disease, rhinitis . . . but there was nothing much I could do about it besides taking my meds. "And don't worry," he patted me reassuringly on the shoulder. "You'll get off prednisone and your clothes will fit you again."

*Grrr.*

On the way out of his office, I ran into a fellow Wegener's patient. She was one of the support group organizers, a lovely woman my age who was also trying to develop a career. I liked her and could relate to her. "Hi, Wendy." She spoke in a low, husky voice due to the Wegener's landing in her larynx. It had led to multiple tracheotomies. Her nose had collapsed, too. We chatted for a few, my existential agitation growing as I saw her features mirror my own. Stalking out of the office, I got furious—so pissed I had this stupid fucking disease.

Finally, a well-deserved fistful of disease-related sadness and anger punched me in the kisser. No wonder I had a flat nose. I cried in bed that night feeling sorry for myself, wanting someone to take care of me, yearning for the mother who had died when I was a little girl. I blew my broken-down proboscis and took a breath. I had to grow up, shrink down, and find a relationship. I was too attached to my parents. And clearly I wasn't working hard enough to get rid of this stupid autoimmune disease. There had to be more I could do. I gently massaged my sore knees, hips, shoulders, and elbows. I felt like I was living in some old lady's body. I wished (ludicrously, I know) that the disease were worse, so that I could blame something for my weight and people would know I wasn't fat for lack of willpower.

There was one upside to contracting Wegener's: If I could take on the horrible disease/death, odds were that my friends and family would be safe. Everyone knows someone in his or her generation who died before her time. I could be that person. I could handle it. I didn't have a husband or kids to leave behind. It would be a fitting punishment for the way I'd been wasting my life and destroying my body with too much food and too little care. . . . Ew, that was morbid. Must be the prednisone talking. I would find the energy to turn my life around. Get my body back. Get *me* back. I needed to start crack-a-lackin' on a major life do-over. I'd envision the phenomenal, healthy, self-confident woman I'd planned to become.

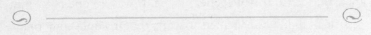

AUGUST 1999

I returned to a building where I swore I'd never show up again, the office of a famous weight loss doctor named Louis Aronne. He was also David Letterman's doctor. Why Dave needed to see a weight loss specialist . . . ? Beyond me. Always obsessed with women's bodies and size (maybe more than we knew), Dave had recently measured Julia Roberts's waist with a tape measure on his show. Twenty-five inches, by the way. Mine was slightly bigger. I weighed in at 258.5. Massive. Probably not Dave's type. After a discussion about my Wegener's complications with Dr. Aronne, I signed up to restart Optifast, that classic diet plan that inspired Oprah to pull around a wagon full of fat and wear supertight jeans. I would drink five- or six-hundred-calorie packets of chocolate-flavored protein powder, two hot cups of bouillon, and two glasses of Metamucil daily for an untold number of weeks until the weight started pouring off. I left the doctor's office and chewed on one final prestarvation Tootsie Roll, idly wondering why lingerie commercials always showed models lounging around, hanging over banisters and running through curtains. Real women are in a *rush*. We have shit to *do*.

At least my deal had gone through. I'd officially signed on to be the editorial director of Oxygen, and the execs were finally talking about the many roles I could fulfill on-air. Anchor, field report, panel host . . . Gerry, the CEO, teasingly asked me how many jobs I was doing for her. I was relieved that only she knew that I had this Wegener's thing. It was no one else's business, and I didn't want staffers to worry that it would compromise my dedication and energy. The workload was beginning to flip me out with stress—short temper here, no sleep there—but was *sooo* worth it.

Coincidentally, one of my coworkers was Charlotte, a producer I'd worked with at MTV. I'd always remembered her because she was smart, loved movies, and happened to be pals with

Madonna, my beyond-favorite entertainer. On her way out of the Oxygen office one night, Charlotte poked her head in my cube. "Wendy, want to come out to dinner?"

I still had to write content guides for all the new shows, go over scripts for an online animation series, and read through thick packets of research that could help us fine-tune our promotional campaigns to appeal to our audience of underserved female TV viewers. I also had to pack up and move desks—again. Our workforce was growing. I could barely walk due to my joint pain, and it wasn't like I was going to suck down an Optifast shake in front of a table full of new colleagues instead of eating a meal . . . "I wish I could," I told her, "but I'm too busy."

"Too bad," she sang, skipping down the stairs. "It's going to be a Ciccone event!"

Missing dinner with Madonna? Damn me.

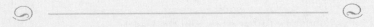

SEPTEMBER 1999

When I went to my checkup with Turner the next week (never a week went by without appointments), he had excellent news: "Looks like you are in clinical remission." That's it? It's over? Maybe the symptoms would finally start fading away. What a dream, to move without pain. A day without a nosebleed. How did I get so lucky? I'd been making the Wegener's a bigger deal than it was, using it as an excuse or to get sympathy. *Thank you, thank you . . . .*

Thank who?

You know, you. God. The Universe. Whatever accounted for my thoughts when I closed my eyes and prayed. I didn't have the specifics down when it came to faith. I wanted to believe that there was something bigger than me, or a motivation for our lives that went beyond biology. When we were little, Mick played a recording of *The 2000 Year Old Man* for Josh and me. Mel Brooks played the 2000 Year Old Man with an old-school Yiddish accent, and Carl Reiner interviewed him as the straight man. Besides *The Muppet Show*, it was the first comedy influence I had—classic Borscht Belt, witty, semi-improvised Jewish outsider humor. In the sequel, *2000 & 13*, Reiner asks the Old Man if ancient people believed in the Almighty.

INTERVIEWER: Did you believe in anything?

OLD MAN: Yes, a guy—Phil. Philip was the leader of our tribe.

INTERVIEWER: What made him the leader?

OLD MAN: Very big, very strong, big beard, big arms, he could just kill you. He could walk on you and you would die.

INTERVIEWER: You revered him?

OLD MAN: We prayed to him. Would you like to hear one of our prayers? "Oh, Philip. Please don't take our eyes out and don't pinch us and don't hurt us. . . . Amen."

INTERVIEWER: How long was his reign?

OLD MAN: Not too long. Because one day, Philip was hit by lightning. And we looked up and said . . . "There's something bigger than Phil!"

I'd stick with that. I didn't have the answers, but I knew there was something BTP: bigger than Phil.

When I went back to the weight loss clinic to officially kick off my final hard-core diet, I was 257.2 on the scale. That was it. I didn't have time to go to Duke. But finally I was going to do it for real, take it one day at a time. I wouldn't have to fast forever. I'd focus on the first two weeks and go from there. Yikes, two weeks was a long time. Okay, one week. Seven days. Even if I could survive the first couple of days without screwing up, I'd nail it. I didn't want people at work to know I was actively trying to lose weight. If I didn't drop the pounds, I'd be a failure. If I messed up and ate real food, everyone would know (I was the anti-Kirstie Alley, who screamed about weight loss to any press outlet who would listen—me, I didn't want to be accountable to anyone). I hoped that if I could keep the protein powder regime under wraps, then I could pretty much starve myself for as long as it took me to lose the weight, about eighty pounds. I imagined skipping into the small office cafeteria, pouring a packet of Optifast powder into my plastic Optifast shaker, adding cold water from the cooler, jiggling the cup, and having to explain why I was drinking a cup of brown, half-dissolved water instead of eating a sandwich or a bowl of soup from the stand downstairs for lunch. I could just be bold and say, "I'm on a diet. Fuck off." Hmm, if I got discovered, that sounded like a decent solution.

Two days later I emceed a feminist benefit where Gloria Steinem said hi to me and Joan Osborne played "What If God

Was One of Us" on acoustic guitar. It was another rough night for me. For someone in "clinical remission," I still had terrible pain in my left leg. It started in my thigh and shot all the way down to my foot. My gums felt swollen and sore. I ignored the pain while I performed, but I'm sure it wasn't my best set. Plus my left eyelid looked all swollen and funky because it had ripped open during that recent brow wax with Olga; my skin was now paper thin due to the side effects of the medication. I had the good sense not to let the wax woman at my right brow, but my face looked lopsided. At least the Optifast was going okay. I'd only eaten five packets that day and the day before, along with two cups of hot bouillon and a Metamucil chaser. I longed for real chow. The next week I went to the clinic and weighed in at 248, down almost eleven pounds. But I did not feel elated about the loss. I felt hungry.

Despite my private self-loathing, my superiors locked in an offer: I would host and produce Oxygen's live daily show, *Pure Oxygen*. It was happening! My TV-hosting dream! I celebrated that weekend with all my favorite people: talked to Sam and Emmy, did brunch and a MAC makeup run with Joe. Randy called. I had coffee at Bret's with Joe and his boyfriend, John, met up with Marybeth and Tami, came back to my place and watched Barbra Streisand suffer in *The Way We Were*, then watched my new favorite show, *Felicity*. I once again added the appetite suppressant Meridia to the Optifast as a backup plan. The drug was expensive, but surely not more expensive than the meals I wasn't eating. I hoped the Meridia wouldn't counteract any of the Wegener's meds, but I honestly didn't care. By my next weigh-in, I'd lost another 13.2 pounds, for a monthlong total of thirty-two.

At work, we were about to shift into our new studio and office space. Oprah, one of our major investors, planned to drop in the following week; I hoped I'd get a chance to meet and greet her (I practiced not fawning in the mirror). In addition to all of that, Gerry tasked me with the biggest creative challenge of them all: to rethink some less-than-fabulous Super Bowl spots that would air a week before the channel launch. I was unsure about our ad campaign, "Another great reason to be a woman." It felt kind of deprecatory and vague. During the few hours I slept, I dreamed about Tom Cruise and Nicole Kidman. Going on ten years together, and they said it wouldn't last! Everything felt full of potential.

When we finally finished taping the *Pure Oxygen* pilots (two versions—one straight and one silly, which was the version I preferred), I had mixed emotions. I felt my hosting performance was fairly strong, but I had lots to learn. Plus it took huge energy to be ebullient on air and keep up all the positive vibes with the crew while we shot—which I thought was essential to doing a good job on the show. It was challenging to think as both producer and talent . . . but how cool to finally be the talent! To get the hair! The makeup! The wardrobe! The attention! The laughs! I was doing exactly what was meant to be, slimming down and achieving remission. Good-bye, Wegener's. Farewell, fat. I was on my way.

# 3

# Keep It Together

DECEMBER 6, 1999

MY 28TH BIRTHDAY

**CURRENT FAVORITE TV SHOW:**
*Should be Buffy spin-off* Angel, *but David Boreanaz was
never my favorite part of the show. Big silent studs
never do it for me. Speaking of studs . . .*

**CURRENT FAVORITE MOVIE:**
*Hoping it will be Brad Pitt's* Fight Club, *because it was
directed by David Fincher, who did Madonna's
"Express Yourself" video*

**CURRENT CRAVING:**
*Swedish Fish, but only the red ones*

**IN MADONNA NEWS:**
*Her Anglophilia escalates as she plans to school
Lourdes in the U.K.*

The indispensible tabloid paper the *New York Post* was
always surprisingly accurate with my horoscope. On
my twenty-eighth birthday, the year's forecast read:
"You will care even less than usual what other people think about

you this year, and some of the things you do will cause a certain amount of shock. Partners and colleagues may say you are acting outrageously, but you're not, you're just ahead of your time."

According to astrologers, your twenty-eighth birthday ushers in a period called Saturn Returns, when the ringed planet shows up in the same position it was in when you were born (also known as "a quarterlife crisis"). It forces you to stop, rethink, and assess your place in life. I assessed away: A year earlier I'd been sick, but had no idea I had an autoimmune disease. I'd worked my weight down to 228. To be semihealthy now felt lucky, like maybe I escaped the wrathful pointy finger of an angry God. I was grateful for the love and support of my circle of friends. I prayed for the health and happiness of my parents and brother, my living grandmothers and extended family, my friends and coworkers. I thought wistfully of my mother, the grandfathers and grandma I loved and lost. Even our dog, Inky, who was currently buried in a Jewish pet cemetery outside Detroit, next to a bulldog named Matzo Ball Friedman. Y2K loomed. If we made it into a new millennium, I hoped we'd make the most of it. That's surely what I needed to do in my twenty-eighth year. *Make the most of it.*

Then . . . kiss that optimism good-bye. I got dropped from the show. They still wanted me as a writer and producer, but not as host. Roni, the executive producer, had always been supportive of me—when she noticed I was losing weight, she said, "Good for you, but don't feel like you have to do it for us." She told me the bad news privately, and then shared it with the rest of the staff. I couldn't stop crying; I scrambled out of the building to avoid conversations and humiliation. I went to a screening of *Magnolia* in

Midtown. There's a movie to lift your spirits. Shit. I still had some on-air options, according to the higher-ups. I could shoot some field segments for *Pure Oxygen*, and they wanted to use my hosting skills on an Internet shopping show called *She-Commerce*. As if. Who would buy goods on a computer when you could waltz right into a store?

When I returned to work the following day, the show staff was shocked at my dismissal and hugely supportive of me. Marta, my co-comedienne, was my shoulder to cry on. Producers and crew members pulled me aside to encourage me, "You are great!" Then Gerry called to explain, "You are *loved*. You are a mega talent. We just want to take the show in a different direction." What direction? The direction of *not* mega talent? I felt so protective of Oxygen and invested in it, this source of entertainment and information for women that didn't talk down to us or reduce us to lowest-common-denominator stereotypes. Gerry had given us a mandate to change the world, and I was sure we could do it. If I wasn't talented enough, not destined for on-air greatness, I hoped she would simply be honest with me so I could stop wasting my time. I was so tired. My bones hurt. My eyes were swollen. I hungered for real human food that didn't come in a packet—but at least when I returned to the office that day after my dismissal, I was wearing size 16 pants.

I stalked around the block in the industrial downtown neighborhood near the studio, feeling sad, silly, and embarrassed. Why had I let myself get so devoted to a TV network? It wasn't going to love me back. It wasn't my name on the door. What made me think I was safe? So foolish of me. It ended like every job, every relationship: I assumed things were going famously, then rug—pull—me—floor. I knew my pattern: I'd fume for a while, and then make a plan. I could take what the network offered, host this other shopping show . . . write cultural criticism for a magazine . . . leave the network and do more comedy . . . Uch uch uch. Watching the new hosts start shooting *Pure Oxygen* made me burn. Gerry tried to soften the blow by inviting me to her home in Telluride over Christmas to surprise Emmy. It hurt. Take a breath. Think.

*I am so frustrated.*

*I can't bend my knees.*

*I am sad.*

*I keep dreaming about hotels.*

*I am lonely.*

*I always feel guilty.*

*I can never get my body fully back.*

*I have no idea how to live in my body.*

*I don't know what I'm supposed to be doing, but I fear I'm not doing it.*

*I wonder where I went wrong . . .*

No, no, you ass. Think positive. Cultivate gratitude, Oprah-style. Okay.

*I can fit into my red jeans.*

*I have red nails.*

*I have soft skin.*

*I have a disease but I think it's getting better.*

*I can't believe my parents are so supportive of me.*

*I am so lucky to have my apartment.*

*I am so lucky to have this life.*

*I wonder when I'll know what I'm meant to do.* My Owen Meany moment.

Better. My goals for the new year: Confidence. Perspective. Perseverance. Less secrecy; more intimacy. Less fear; more faith. Stop picking my cuticles. Send good vibes to J-Lo and Puffy to make it through another paparazzi-fueled month. The calendar shifted from 1999 to 2000 without a moment of Y2K's forecasted digital drama.

---

## JANUARY 2000

A few weeks later I was engrossed in the turmoil of producing and shooting. I was already enamored of my new cohosts and our production team on the Internet shopping show, *She-Commerce*. It was formatted like *The View*, with four different hosts representing four different points of view. I was the plus-size body image rep; Janine was the suburban mom; Leticia was the spicy single Latina; and Sloan was the wealthy, savvy shopper. Instant cohost lovefest. Our studio for our roundtable segments was a Starbucks in Midtown. We drank tons of latte and pounded scones. Not too many—my fighting weight was down to 215, a total of forty-three lost pounds. Days were busy and fun, but nights were awful—I was racked with pain that radiated from my left shoulder and down my arm. I couldn't move and could barely sleep. When I did, I dreamed that Madonna had adopted a bunch of kids from around the world. Yeah, right. I dug up an old bottle of Tylenol with codeine to get a couple of hours of pain-free z's. Sleep was essential—I had full shoot days at Starbucks, plus re-shoots of three green-screen shopping segments from the week before. I worked the red carpet at the National Board of Review and interviewed Clint Eastwood, Sigourney Weaver, and Hilary Swank, who got canned from *90210* and was getting raves for her performance as a girl who wanted to be a boy in *Boys Don't Cry*. Supposedly she'd lost enough weight to get down to 7 percent body fat, which must have all been centered in her boobs. *Harper's Bazaar* featured a story about Oxygen's channel launch, including a big picture of me. The busier things got at work, the more agony I felt. My ANCA antibody level had increased, so I was still popping fifteen milligrams of prednisone each day. Turner was concerned I might also have fibromyalgia, a chronic condition that causes widespread pain in joints and pressure points; he suggested I try Advil to stave off the discomfort. More discomfort? Take more Advil. He was uneasy about prescribing a more intense level of meds that could lead me to drug addiction. My goal was to not take *any* drugs. I really didn't think of myself as the druggie type.

The eve of Oxygen's "birth" day capped off a chaotic, hellish week. The studio/office space was a big, open loft, so the volume level was high-school-freshman-who-just-discovered-Nirvana-loud. I tried to keep a lid on my stress but it kept popping off. I snapped at a wardrobe assistant who wanted me to wear a sleeveless dress. I fumed at the editors who couldn't follow my directions without me sitting next to them in the edit suite. I had to be in ten places at once. The dangling carrot that made it worth the drama: I had scored an interview with Madonna.

*Madonna!* Who was better than that?

Back when I was a budding bat mitzvah girl in Michigan, I was so naïve that I wasn't even sure what *virgin* meant. But Madonna says that according to Kabbalistic teachings, "Thirteen is the age when the soul gets solidified in your body, when you come into your own." Figures that's when I came into Madonna. My Ciccone cherry officially got popped in 1985, when I saw her Virgin Tour concert at Joe Louis Arena in downtown Detroit. I vividly recall her straddling a big boom box while purring, "Every lady has a box." I guess they do, I thought nervously, but I don't know if they hump 'em like that.

Madonna was bold and sexy and Catholic and scary and original and fearless—all things I was *not*. I was nice and sweet and Jewish and terrified of anything boldly sexual. I hated my swollen preteen body and really, really wanted everyone to like me. Still, I felt a bond with the naughty video vixen. We had so much in common. We'd both been raised in the suburbs of Detroit. We were both Daddy's girls who would do anything for his affection and approval. We both liked attention; we were both creative. She was a Leo; I was a Sagittarius—both fire signs. Our deepest connection was that Madonna's mom had died when she was six; I was ten when I lost mine. When my dad remarried, I fell in love with my stepmother. Madonna didn't get so lucky.

In August 1989, when I was seventeen, I bought tickets to see

Madonna's Blond Ambition tour. I was insanely excited to go. I was a college-freshman-to-be (at the University of Michigan, which Madonna had attended and escaped). My friends and I had nosebleed seats at the Pontiac Silverdome (when we saw Bruce Springsteen at the Silverdome in 1984, he got the crowd so pumped that a cloud formed in the pocket of the dome and all our sweat rained back down on us). I remember exactly what I wore to Madonna's concert: a silky, pearlescent silver blouse, flowing silk lavender palazzo pants, and my long strand of fake pearls. From the first note, I was mesmerized. Madonna was a dynamic ball of energy whirling around the stage in a whiplike braid and her infamous cone bra, insisting that we both express ourselves and keep it together at the same time. She was a teeny person, but larger than life to me. When my friends went to get drinks during the *Dick Tracy* section (fine, it wasn't the most exciting part of the show), I refused to leave my seat. I didn't want to miss a minute of the spectacle miles below. Madonna demanded that we sing "Happy Birthday" to her daddy. When I later saw her face in close-up at that moment during the documentary *Truth or Dare*, she beamed. I left that concert Girl-hooked for life.

In college my Madonna fascination continued to grow. I joined the Official Fan Club (member #15489) and stashed the ID card in my wallet. I collected mags and photos; I framed a giant poster of her face from a *Harper's Bazaar* shoot and hung it in my bedroom. Her hair was blond and wet, and she wore a heavy metal necklace of triangles, like a tribal icon watching over me. I couldn't sleep a wink the night before the *Sex* book came out. I'd preordered it from an Ann Arbor record shop and lined up greedily with all the other gay boys and fag hags who had done the same. I ran home to the apartment I shared with Sam on Oakland Street and was shaking as I slit open the silver Mylar package. I flipped the metal cover (which legendarily didn't turn very easily) as if I delicately held the pages of an ancient Bible in my hands . . . yikes. The images confused me, kind of freaked me out. Shaved-headed lesbians menacing Madge in a high school gym. Some German guy stalking around a biker bar. Vanilla Ice. I found the sexuality too in my face. A lot of the text was surprisingly graphic and base. I tried not to read too much into an offhanded remark about fat being "a problem" for Madonna, making her think "'overindulgent pig.'" Still, as a book owner, I became a little bit of a local celeb, luring guys into my bedroom with "Hey, wanna look at my copy of the *Sex* book?"

During this time in the early 1990s, PC feminism stormed college campuses, including my own. My adoration for Madonna was deemed completely in conflict with the Third Wave. Apparently I couldn't Take Back the Night if I didn't also take back my MAC Russian Red lipstick (the kind Madonna wore on tour; when Myrn sent a tube to me at school it was like receiving treasure in the mail). I didn't understand why dismissing sexuality was seen as a positive step for women; wasn't Madonna reinventing the rules? Couldn't we be seductive and feminist at the same time? Couldn't "sex-positive" feminists and "antipornography" feminists find some common ground? My zealous friends borrowed from my treasure trove of Material swag to prove points about her regressive sexual evil for a Feminism 101 class. I didn't buy it. There was something about Madonna that made me feel invulnerable, invincible, acceptable. Whenever I had moments of confusion or doubt, her lyrics reached out to guide me: *Open your heart. Justify my love. Express yourself—so you can respect yourself.*

During my junior year I left Ann Arbor for New York, as Madonna had done in 1978. I did not eat french fries out of the garbage, nor did I pick up skinny Latin guys while cruising around in a limousine on the Lower East Side, as she supposedly did. I attended New York University for a semester, traipsing around the funky streets of the East Village. Living in New York City felt like coming home: the dirt, the noise, the drama, and the danger; people of all colors and shapes and sizes and ages and interests. I got high and hooked up, hit clubs and produced short experimental films. I met new friends, discovered new ideas, and somehow found myself interning at MTV (to my parents' horror), at a time when the most famous bands on the channel were either thick black girls singing about condoms or skinny white boys singing about drugs. In all these years, MTV hasn't changed very much.

I'd promised my folks I would return to Ann Arbor my senior year to finish my degree at Michigan, where I hung my big Madonna poster on my bedroom wall once again. The day after graduation I packed my belongings in our car and began the ten-hour drive to Manhattan, my new home.

The Oxygen interview wouldn't be my first meeting with the Girl. One of my first jobs out of college in the early '90s was working at MTV as an assistant in the celebrity talent department. My job was to coordinate travel for the VJs and occasionally escort C-list celebs to set visits and award shows. "Jenna von Oy from *Blossom*? Right this way!" "Down this hall, Another Bad Creation!" My boss earned my lifelong appreciation one day when she told me she'd arranged for me to be Madonna's liaison at the 1994 Video Music Awards.

Holy erotica! I'd been a massive fan for years, but I realized what had lured me to work at MTV in the first place: I wanted to meet Madonna, and maybe get a personal blessing from the woman I considered to be my spiritual guide. I didn't necessarily think of her as a "guru," but she certainly fit the bill. *Guru* is a Sanskrit word for someone with great wisdom who shares that wisdom with others. A teacher. The syllables of the word referred to darkness (*gu*) and the destroyer of darkness (*ru*), so a guru was someone who could guide you from dark to light. Make the invisible visible. Turn on a spiritual lightbulb.

I met Madonna for the very first time—like a virgin, you might say—at the VMA rehearsals. I wore my limited edition "Girlie Show" tour watch (flip it open and you'd find a condom inside) when I went to greet Ms. Ciccone and her entourage at Radio City Music Hall, where the producers planned to walk her through her paces for the next night's show. I was shaking when I finally came face-to-face with her, a legendary, tiny force of nature. Madonna was so small, barely over five feet tall and surprisingly small-boned, but she had the biggest, bluest eyes I'd ever seen. Her hair was short and blond; her skin practically glowed. Dazzling. She was accompanied by her sexy/juicy New Yawky assistant, Caresse; her confident, mustachioed manager, Freddy; her incredibly hot security guard, Robert; her formidable publicist, Liz Rosenberg; and my producer pal, Charlotte. Charlotte announced, "Wendy is a *huge* fan," pointing out my condom-packed watch. I could have died of embarrassment. But I didn't. Madonna gave a nod of approval, and a slew of producers assaulted her with instructions. In frustration, she turned to me and said, "I want YOU to know everything." I told her I would. In reality, she was ordering me to keep track of the details that would keep the night running smoothly. Now I like to think she was giving me her blessing ("I want you to"), and offering me the wisdom of the world ("Know everything.").

I was determined to make sure nothing marred Madonna's night at the VMAs. She had provided me with so much wisdom; an error-free evening was the least I could offer in return. For example, I knew she didn't like air-conditioning, so I went to her dressing room and unwired it before she arrived. When her makeup artist (some French dame named Laura Mercier) wished aloud that she had additional lights to illuminate Madonna's every pore, I made sure Laura got them. I dumped the Skittles out of Madonna's gift basket and refilled it with her favorite candies: lemon drops, Red Hots, and candy dots on paper (even though she probably hadn't touched them in years). I double-checked to make sure the occupants of the dressing room next door wouldn't disturb her, waking U2's Bono and Adam Clayton from a much-needed nap in the process.

What a night—for me. Madonna showed up with the whole entourage, luscious in a glittery ball gown and Goth *Cabaret* "Secret" look: penciled eyebrows, red lips, short platinum hair in marcelle waves. She had recently sparred with David Letterman by swearing thirteen times on his talk show, and his top-secret cameo was planned for her award presentation. I brushed past

Michael Jackson and Lisa Marie Presley (who opened the show with the world's most awkward mash session) to line up the Spice Girls outside Madonna's door, urging them to calm down as they came to pay their respects. When we took an elevator to the main floor, I made a joke and *Madonna laughed.* My heart sang, "And it feels like . . . hoooo-me." I body-checked Keith Richards and Mick Jagger when they got in Madonna's way backstage. When Madonna decided on the spur of the moment that she wanted to powder her nose, I cleared thirty women out of a public bathroom—insisting a security guard carry an enraged and screaming VH1 executive VP out of the room. At one point, Madonna didn't feel like going up to the Radio City Music Hall marquee at the time she was scheduled for an interview. The executive producers of the VMAs jumped out of the director's truck to hunt me down and order me to make Madonna go where she needed to go. "Make" Madonna do something she didn't want to do? Ha! I jumped so far up their grills that I could have plucked their vocal cords, one by one, insisting resolutely, "Madonna is gonna go wherever *she* wants to go, whenever *she* wants to get there!" I was a lowly twenty-one-year-old talent assistant, but they were so shocked that they turned around and skulked back into the truck. Liz Rosenberg, whom I feared and adored, was totally impressed. For the next several MTV events, she insisted that I serve as Madonna's talent liaison.

So I was on the red carpet the following year when Courtney Love chucked her MAC makeup compact at a Gucci-clad, high-ponytailed Madonna while the latter chatted with Kurt Loder at the VMAs. I was on the scene when Madonna read a children's book (long before the days she was writing them herself) to a nightclub crowd while wearing silk pajamas. And I witnessed the best moment of all, when Madonna and Sean Penn saw each other for the first time since their divorce, in the middle of all the mayhem at the first VH1/Vogue Fashion Awards. The instant they laid eyes on each other, it was as though they stood still in the center of a tornado. Like that scene in *West Side Story* when the other gang members freeze around Tony and Maria, then slip out in the middle of the dance at the gym. The world swirled around Madonna and Sean, but they were locked on each other: The contact between them was completely and totally still. I have never seen two people connect so deeply in such a brief moment. That image and feeling have stayed with me forever: *Ah, so* that's *what love is supposed to look like.* It's been awfully hard to find.

Later that night, Madonna's manager asked me if I wanted to interview for a position at Maverick, Madonna's fledgling production company. You bet I did. The next day at the St. Regis hotel, I totally bombed the interview. I couldn't stop sweating; it turns out her manager wasn't a fan of air-conditioning, either. I wore glasses to look smarter; he asked me, "Do you really need to wear glasses, or are you just wearing them to look smarter?" I followed up with him when he returned to L.A., but he didn't respond to my inquiries. So Hollywood. Eventually I left my full-time talent job at MTV to pursue my own writing and producing career. Still, my passion for Madonna, and my spiritual belief and material support for all of her endeavors, never waned.

With the help of my friend Joe, another Madonna fanatic

dressed in MTV executive clothing, we chased the Girl around the globe, hitting concerts, collecting music and DVDs, sharing websites. It wasn't just the music and the spectacle that enticed me; at every show I saw—and I saw many—I would look forward to the instant when I would feel a mysterious rush, a private moment of enlightenment as if Madonna were personally tapping a wand to my forehead (also known as the third eye, or sixth chakra, a place of illumination). I never knew when to expect it; the energy never touched me during the same song twice. Now, as a TV correspondent for Oxygen, I was going to meet with her face-to-face, as a professional broadcaster.

m-Day. Madonna Day. I blew up at office staffers who crossed in front of my camera line on their way to the bathroom (why they built a camera studio in between the office and the bathroom is still beyond me), and cried in my dressing room. Then I scooted out of the office to meet up with Madonna.

Madonna—sure, I'd believe it when I was in the room for our interview. I frantically waved down a cab on Tenth Avenue. I'd only been given four minutes to talk with the icon about her latest movie. Bet Diane Sawyer got six minutes. Whatever—all I got was four minutes to save the world. The flick she was promoting was *The Next Best Thing.* You remember (or maybe you don't): the one where she played a yoga instructor who wanted to have a baby by herself with her gay best friend, played by Rupert Everett—yeah, yeah.

That workday, like every one preceding it, had been insanely busy. The network planned to launch that day, and I'd barely have time to attend the party to celebrate it. Once I finished the interview, I'd have to run back to the office, recut the package, finish the next day's scripts, set up another edit . . . cool by me. It was worth the stress to have my first face-to-face interview with Madonna.

I tried to pick out an outfit that would flatter me, but my options were minimal. I was so big. It wasn't just fat that threw me off—the steroids I'd been taking for a year had Jiffy Popped my body. They were supposed to stop inflammation, relieving swelling and pain, but my joints were still killing me. I was still doing that supervised medical fast to try to counteract the steroid weight gain. My personality vacillated between "starving psycho" and "raving lunatic."

I made it to the lobby of the Regency Hotel, where I waited with all the other media hoity-toits. I recognized correspondents from *Entertainment Tonight* and *Access Hollywood*. Could I really make a career out of this? Fat or sick or not, I was about to interview my idol in a segment that would eventually air on a show I hosted on a new network that I'd help create. I scanned my list of questions for the umpteenth time. Should I have fun with her? Be a serious journalist? Would she and her team remember me from the MTV days?

A production assistant with a clipboard called out, "Wendy Shanker?"

I stood up, straightened my dress (a brown velvet Eileen Fisher A-line that I'd recently worn to my cousin's bar mitzvah in Detroit) and my necklace (a vintage piece I grabbed out of Myrn's jewelry box), and slipped past the tables of fruit and old cheese that had been set out hours ago for the press. Liz and Caresse remembered me and greeted me warmly; the foxy bodyguard, Robert, did, too (he'd been working for Janet Jackson and went on to guard Jennifer Lopez). Madonna's on-and-off frenemy Ingrid Casares lingered in the background. I slipped past an exiting Matt Lauer and into the chair, still warm with Lauer tush.

The interview was the fastest three minutes of my life (four minutes had been downgraded to three before I arrived). Madonna wore a casual blue top, her hair long, blond, and curly. She seemed more relaxed to me this time—maybe she was so exhausted by all the interviews that she didn't have the energy to keep her defensive celebrity shield up and running. She looked angelic, had a glow around her face. Sonya Dakar oxygen facial or happiness? You decide. I didn't know it then, but she was pregnant with her second child, Rocco.

As she acknowledged me, I saw a gleam of recognition in Madonna's bottomless blue eyes. A producer clicked a stopwatch to start the three-minute countdown, and Madonna conspiratorially leaned forward to whisper something in my ear. "Go ahead," she told me. "Be brilliant."

Whoa. She'd given me an order to be brilliant, to say something incredibly smart and unforgettable. About a yoga movie. In three minutes. I didn't know if I could meet the challenge. The stopwatch clicked ominously. A cameraman rolled his eyes as I hesitated. Then I realized, Madonna wasn't *telling* me to be brilliant. She was giving me *permission*.

Guru power activated!

I shot the interview, chatted about the movie, and made Madonna chuckle. I don't know if I'd officially classify it as "brilliant," but I felt like I had almost saved the world. I rushed back for a toast at the Oxygen launch party, but my buzz only lasted for a few minutes. I had to write scripts, screen segments of a movie with Ben Affleck and Charlize Theron, prep interviews with my comedy inspirations Sandra Bernhard and Tracey Ullman . . . .There was work to be done. I scowled at my coworkers on what was supposed to be a triumphant day, stomped back to my desk, and strapped on giant headphones to block out the party noise.

When I look back on the Oxygen era, I can see that my behavior was spiraling wildly out of control. I was working with no sleep. On steroids. In pain. Secretly sick. Sneaking opiates. Starving. Doing twelve jobs. Hosting live TV shows. Having zero social life. Trying desperately to fulfill the mandate that had been given to me to make the world a better place for women, and impress Gerry, my role model. I don't know the equivalent of going postal at a TV network, but I was probably close. I knew I had to get my temper, anger, and bad attitude under control.

There had to be a better way. WWMD? What would Madonna do? Probably start her own network. Slamming doors in frustration made me look like an idiot. It accomplished nothing. One of my best friends, Deb, had a vivacious cousin I adored named Amy. Amy had just been diagnosed with melanoma. *That* was a real problem. What did I have to complain about? I also began to notice that after every blowup, I'd be in more pain. I had pain shooting in my left hand, up to the elbow on my right arm. I was always constipated or sick to my stomach. Because I was a human being who needed food, I started eating again. I couldn't breathe. During the few hours I slept, I had nightmares.

I returned to the weight loss clinic. Down only one pound, to 214. Dr. Aronne saw me glowering on the scale and urged me to calm down. "Are you under a lot of stress?" he asked.

"Oh, just a bit," I sneered.

"I'm not surprised. Stress does the same thing to the body that prednisone does," he explained. "It releases the hormone cortisol in the system, which is often called the stress hormone. You feel a rush of it in response to stress and anxiety. It increases blood pressure, raises blood sugar, and shuts down your immune system. That's why doctors prescribe prednisone, which is essentially synthetic cortisone, to treat autoimmune diseases; it controls your immune system so it won't work overtime. But it's like having bursts of adrenaline pump through your system twenty-four hours a day. Prednisone and excess cortisol can also make your insulin level rise." That imbalance would eventually cause my body to become insulin resistant, aka diabetic. Ah, insulin. Years of attempted weight loss had given me a full background on that subject. I knew that the pancreas releases insulin to process simple carbohydrates; when that signal gets screwed up, your body does, too. The more carbs you eat, the more carbs you crave. Bigger appetite, less satiation, more weight gain. Plus prednisone clearly made me hyper and mean, and impaired my judgment. I couldn't stay this stressed-out, I wouldn't leave my job, and I couldn't stay on prednisone forever. But my docs had no other options to offer me. For my own sanity and the safety of others, I would have to figure out short- and long-term cortisol-free solutions.

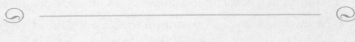

MARCH 2000

I woke up one morning and couldn't move my elbow. It was swollen, warm to the touch, and it *hurt*. To be awakened by pain indicated to me that something was really wrong. This wasn't a "little, yellow, Nuprin" situation; Turner's advice to take Advil wasn't going to cut it, either. I snuck out of work to show him the puffy elbow joint that was preventing me from sitting at my desk or bending my arms.

Dr. Turner examined the elbow, which now looked seriously inflamed and slightly bruised. I whimpered when he tried to bend it. He mused aloud, "This might be a buildup of uric acid, which could indicate gout."

Rheumy-eyed old men in Dickens tales often suffered from gout! Rheum strikes again! Add it to the list. Wegener's, fibromyalgia, now gout . . . Turner pulled out a long needle so that he could take a sample of the fluid in the joint, and delivered that infamous Western medical understatement: "This might hurt a little."

The prick-'n'-pull did way more than hurt. Gooey fluid that looked like chicken fat spurted out of my elbow, spraying Dr. Turner's white coat and even hitting the wall. It was so disgusting, but for a gunk-and-dismemberment fan like me (I TiVo *Trauma: Life in the ER*), it was perversely exciting. Dr. Turner almost lost his composure calling for help while trying to suck the rest of the gunk out of my arm. After I was cleaned up and bandaged, we left the exam room and sat down in his office. Diplomas decorated the walls; every surface except for his chair and mine was covered with paperwork, scans, and patient folders. Turner cleared his throat and said, "Wendy, that elbow must have really been hurting you. That situation required more than Advil. I want to apologize for underestimating your pain. It won't happen again." I could understand making a mistake; I have no tolerance for someone who can't admit he made one. Turner's apology solidified my trust in him. I thought to myself, If anyone can fix me, it's this guy.

That night the moon hung low in the sky, clear after days of rain. I woke up again in the middle of the night, but not from elbow juice. I heard a voice in my head say, "Let go . . ." like the tail end of a dream. Whose voice? Bigger Than Phil's voice? An utterance from the great beyond? Some maniac screaming below my window on Seventy-second Street? I flipped on the light at my bedside table and peeled back the curtain. No crazy homeless guy shouting, no drunk girl giggling on her way in or out of a cab. The voice somehow came from inside me.

I climbed back into bed and left the light on. Should I be concerned that I was hearing voices, or open myself up to the possibility that my intuition was providing me with some direction? "Let go." The problem was, I didn't know what exactly to let go of. Control? Concern? Or like "Let go and be done," kind of in the "get over it" zone? Guess it was whatever was holding me back, making me crazy, and preventing me from feeling better. I fell back to sleep hearing:

*Let go. Let go. Let go. . . .*

---

OCTOBER 2000

ood news from Turner: My ANCA had dropped to a very low positive. Negative couldn't be far away! My urine showed bacteria and white blood cells, but no blood or protein. And I was only taking four milligrams of prednisone a day—hardly any. Some doctors said anything less than ten milligrams a day wouldn't trip my system; I knew that my body was a lot more sensitive than that. I'd been quaking in my Doc Martens, thinking that if my symptoms didn't get better I'd have to go on Cytoxan, the really scary chemo drug. Now I felt relieved, and celebrated by watching the last few episodes of *The West Wing* and prepping for my trip to L.A. to shoot on the red carpet for the Oscars. Again an odd sense of disappointment percolated—God, don't strike me down—that things weren't worse. Like I wanted people to feel bad for me. Discomforting, since pity had never been my strong suit.

When my mom died, there was no survival and recovery handbook. The assumption was, "Wendy's a strong girl, she can take care of herself." To the naked eye, I did seem to move on and take the loss in stride. I ran for sixth-grade class president. Even I thought I was fine, and I was very pleased to make things easy for my grieving family. But honestly? I was ten! Ten-year-old girls—no matter how mature, how smart, how well mannered—can't handle that shock on their own. Now, at twenty-eight, I felt like a little girl again, but this time I wanted someone to take care of me. The past year had been so rewarding: I got to develop creative ideas and watch them come to fruition, interview celebrities, step in front of the camera. But it had been so disappointing in other ways—the daily physical challenges, the sense that I was way more invested in the channel than the channel was in me. I was tired of doing my life by myself. I needed to speed ahead, move on, plug in, say no to all the negativity and anger, and figure out a way to succeed without screaming, swearing, fighting, or blowing up, mentally or physically. In other words . . . let go.

Ohhh.

But I still required some spiritual support.

I believe that God (or whatever) speaks to you in a language you understand. If the Spirit in the Sky comes down and says, "Le Dieu, c'est moi!" but you don't parlez Français, you're not going to get it. You don't notice symbols and signs, even if you're looking for them, until they show up in your idiom. For example, I speak fluent Madonna. If I get in a fight with a coworker, walk away wondering if I was in the wrong, then go to Sephora and hear "Human Nature" on the sound system (*I'm not your bitch / Don't hang your shit on me*)—that's a sign I was right. See? God may have been chatting with you for a long time, and you just didn't know it! Anyway, I got a sign in a language I could comprehend when we were shooting a *She-Commerce* episode with Gloria Gaynor, singer of "I Will Survive." When Josh and I were little, our mom made us bag lunches—usually tuna fish or PBJ, with a piece of fruit—to take to Jewish Community Center day camp. She'd write our names on them with slim Magic Markers. Some days she'd add a little drawing or doodle. On the day we had a disco dance planned at camp, my mom drew a vinyl record on my lunch bag. The song on the record label? "I Will Survive." She picked it for me because I was a klutz, but twenty-odd years later, dancing around a Starbucks with Gloria Gaynor herself, it felt like a message my mom was sending my way: Be strong, Wendy.

Determined survival would be my theme song.

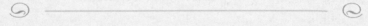

## NOVEMBER 2000

madonna switched to full-on "Music" mode, wearing sparkly cowgirl outfits on *Letterman*. She did a few small exclusive shows to hype the upcoming album. Joe and Bret somehow scored tix to see her at a Midtown club called Roseland. We were *thisclose* to her. The crowd was crazy amped and sweaty. She only played five songs from "Music" (no greatest hits), but she dazzled with her "Beautiful Stranger" hair and a bedazzled cowgirl T-shirt with a glitter iron-on that read BRITNEY SPEARS. The shirt was slit on the sides to make room for her post-Rocco belly. Right, she'd been pregnant when I interviewed her in February. Her daughter, Lourdes was at the show, along with pals Rosie, Donatella, and

Ingrid (as always). Gwyneth waved to the audience from the bal-
cony, like a princess. I glanced up at her when Madonna played
"What It Feels Like for a Girl." Gwyneth was genuinely singing
her heart out, just like me. We might have more in common than
I thought.

T urner asked me to join a trial for a drug called Enbrel. It
was a protein that blocked the body from making a sub-
stance that ordered increased action in the immune system, and
was used to treat rheumatoid arthritis and severe psoriasis. I was
finally part of a scientific experiment! I had to inject the vials into
my thighs twice a week, like a junkie. Soon bruises that looked
like little purple clouds dotted my lap. I felt that old, now trusty
pang of guilt—worried (and grateful) that I hadn't earned the
right to have access to a drug that could help me without hurting
me. Certainly there were other people who needed it more than
me. But who knew? There was only a fifty-fifty chance that I was
even getting Enbrel and not a placebo. I wouldn't know for three
years, when the trial ended. I signed a document promising I
wouldn't get pregnant for three years; I didn't want to give birth
to a Gila monster. Pregnancy was a major option to give up.
Maybe it was worth it. Maybe the Enbrel/not Enbrel would ease
my arthritic pain. No matter what, the study would definitely
help the next guy, so at least I was doing something Good Samar-
itan-ish. I figured if scientists could crack the genomic code
(which they'd recently done—President Clinton called it "God's

code for us"), some genius could certainly come up with a drug to help the over twenty million and growing number of people like me who suffered from autoimmune diseases.

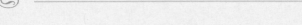

DECEMBER 6, 2000

MY 29TH BIRTHDAY

**CURRENT FAVORITE COUPLE:**
*Britney & Justin (since Ben & Gwyneth are
just hyping it up for a movie)*

**CURRENT FAVORITE TV SHOW:**
The West Wing *(must stop crying at the end
of every episode)*; Alias

**CURRENT BURNING QUESTION:**
*Will Bush or Gore win this election?*

**CURRENT LOOK:**
*Not a thong, no matter how many times they play that
damn Sisqó song*

**IN MADONNA NEWS:**
*Wedding rumors to Guy Ritchie afoot*

A year earlier, my horoscope declared that people would think I was acting "outrageously," but I was simply ahead of my time. Looking ahead to 2001 it read: "Make sure you communicate clearly and simply, both in your personal life and at work. If people know what you expect of them, they will deliver the right thing at the right time and everyone will be happy. If not, chaos rules." But I wasn't feeling solid enough to communicate clearly on my twenty-ninth birthday. Dressing for a birthday dinner with my friends, I thought my low energy could be due to a recent prednisone taper—sometimes even the tiniest shift down in my intake made me feel like I had the flu, and cranked up the joint pain. Or it could be due to a Wegener's flare. Oh, crap. If you get sick, does that mean that God's just not that into you? Maybe I wouldn't even make it as far as thirty-five, like my mom did. Then what did I have to show for my life? Lots of nice stuff, family, friends, laughter, entertainment . . . I had created some good work, but so what? Sixty people had just been laid off from Oxygen. I didn't long to see Paree, I didn't yearn to help the homeless. On the upside, I couldn't wait for my friend Deb's twins to be born. Her cousin Amy was also brimming with anticipation. Cancer or not, she planned to be there to help Deb and her husband, Michael, with the newborns. What if I wanted kids? I had to wait at least three years for true love to inseminate me, or else I'd give birth to an Enbrel mutant. I had put on four pounds, up to 219, so obviously I didn't want love badly enough to keep the weight off. My apathy was so lame, especially when I thought about Amy, who was fighting rapidly spreading melanoma. I was wasting time. Who knew, I could meet the man of my dreams at my birthday dinner. I could have kids if I waited out this experiment and my ovaries didn't fry. Or I could always adopt. But what gave me joy *now*? Where was my passion? What did I love?

Then there was "Why?" A question my doctors couldn't answer. I drove myself crazy trying to figure out why I had Wegener's. One unsettling issue I couldn't completely dismiss: that this was somehow my *fault*. Was I sick from biology, attitude, or God? Could medicine repair my body, or was it up to me to heal the crisis in my soul?

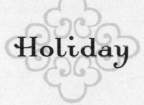

# 4

# Holiday

MARCH 2001

I've often been told that I was supposed to learn some kind of cosmic lesson from the bad things in life. If you are too needy, you discover how to fend for yourself. Or if you are too stubborn, you'll be forced to give up control. As a person who does not like, want, or need help, my mission was to learn how to accept help. For example, two of my closest friends, Tracy and Samantha, were not satisfied with the slow and unsteady results from my Wegener's treatment. They also knew I was overdoing it at work. Intervention time!

I met Tracy and Sam at the University of Michigan. Sam was my next-door-mate in my soul-sucking dorm. She was smart and saucy, had good linens on her bed and a bulimic roommate who booted daily into a bucket that she didn't even bother to hide. Sam introduced me to Tracy, her childhood friend from summer camp. When Sam took a Silicon Valley gig after graduation, she and Tracy moved in together in an apartment in Haight-Ashbury. Tracy was an artist whose work explored transformation, sacred space, nature and the feminine divine. It spoke to my curiosity about those subjects.

Watching me ebb and flow under conventional Western medical care, Tracy and Sam were convinced that I needed unconventional treatment. Easy to say when you're not the patient. I knew the drugs were making my body toxic, but I refused to dismiss the instructions of my medical team. It was too risky. Sure, maybe if I chewed on a banana root and tapped my toes three times under the full moon, I'd heal instantly. But just in case, I was going to pop poisonous pills and sit still for plenty of radioactive CT scans, thank you very much.

Tracy did her best to nudge me towards alternative remedies by sending me organic pain relief tablets and books like *Prescription for Nutritional Healing*. I had never even taken a yoga class, let alone explored nutritional supplements and meditation. I was still reluctant to accept the concept that emotional angst had manifested my physical problems, a tenet of many spiritually based healing plans. When Tracy offered to join me at a spa or alternative healing center, I gave in. But I set up some ground rules:

- **Wherever we went, there could be no screen doors.** Screen doors reminded me of summer camp, and not in a good way. I still jump when I hear the slap of wood against wood.
- **No ladies with long gray braids who refuse to wear makeup and who listen to Joni Mitchell all the time.** I

call them Gray Braiders, women who wear their defiance against beauty the same way plastic surgery addicts try to defy time with a scalpel. I could just picture women gathering in unitards, joining together in matriarchal circles of strength while I sat in the mess hall, wishing I could dump them all in a big vat of Clairol.

- **No traveling to some tropical island or coastal situation.** The sweat factor was a big one for me. I can't emphasize how sweaty I was at the time: 24/7. Always too hot and never comfortable. It could be the middle of December and I'd somehow still get prickly heat.

I wanted to establish every safeguard to avoid becoming one of "those" people, who start out normal-to-rough, then get sick and hear the call, then change their names to "Karma Collins" or "Lotus McGee," do a lot of sun salutations, and drink copious amounts of flaxseed oil. It was important to me to stay New Yorky rotten. This illness wasn't going to change the essential me, dammit.

Tracy generously accepted my parameters. An article called "Detoxing in Kitchari Heaven" miraculously appeared on her radar during her search, and she mailed it to me. It was from the November/December 2000 issue of *Healing Retreats* magazine (until that point, I had no idea such a magazine existed). The author wrote about her experience doing *panchakarma* (PK) at a place called the Ayurvedic Center, in New Mexico, and described the treatment:

"[It] has been used in India for thousands of years to cleanse and rejuvenate the body, mind and consciousness. It is perhaps the most evolved system of detoxification known, involving several techniques: *snehan* (light oil massage), *swedan* (sweating), *shirodhara* (third-eye oil treatment), *nasya* (nasal cleansing), enemas, purgation and emetics, along with the mono-diet of *kitchari*: basmati rice and mung dahl (a kind of lentil)."

I could hear screen doors slamming in my head. The words *enema* and *purgation* twanged deep in my fear lobe. All those Sanskrit italics made me nervous, too. But the author offered up another detail about PK that caught my eye: "It is also deeply calming. Sessions can be emotional, where tears, laughter, and even visions of past lives may surface and be released." Past lives? I'd always been fascinated by that concept. I assumed I'd been, like, Field Worker No. 2 in a past life. Nothing cool, like Amazonian warrior queen, or emperor's favored concubine. Reincarnation was worth exploring. Maybe I'd get more info about how to "let go."

The holdup was that in most health scenarios, I always ended up challenging whoever was in charge. If all those Indian people were all nice and gentle with me, I wouldn't have anyone to tussle with. Luckily, I found a thorn as the writer interviewed Dr. Achari Rai, the founder of the center. When asked why autoimmune diseases are so prevalent, he said, "Autoimmune diseases are nothing but lack of self-esteem and the accumulation of mental *ama* (toxins) in the cells. Your body is attacking itself. Your cells go against themselves and lose their intelligence and attach to similar neighboring cells. And some people get so depressed, they kill themselves. Ayurveda says sin—if you want to accept the concept of sin—is not loving oneself. Not having self-esteem is the biggest sin. But once you learn about your true value in life, then your life becomes a celebration."

Was Dr. Rai suggesting that I got sick because of *low self-esteem?* Oh, it's so on.

Because of my medical situation, the center required me to get a release form from my doctor. I cringe as I think of having sent Turner this note so early in our medical courtship:

*February 5, 2001*

*Dr. Turner:*

*In March, I will be going to a retreat in New Mexico with a friend to do some alternative health stuff (massage, yoga, cleansing diet, etc.). One of the treatments is called Panchakarma. It's the Ayurvedic system of dripping oil on the "third eye" to help rid the body of toxins. It's more extreme than a regular old trip to the spa, and a little bit crazy, but I figure, why the hell not? Still, I need a doctor's permission to do it. Wondering if you would write me a note. (This is like high school gym class.) I can give you more specific info or you can check their website at www.ayurveda.com.*

*Feel free to call me on my cell phone in regards to the above.*

*Thanks,*
*Wendy Shanker*

"OMG, Dr. Turner, will you write me a note? No, not because I need to get out of gym 'cause I have my period. You see, I have to go to a clinic to have my past lives released so I won't have Wegener's anymore." He must have thought I was nuts, but he signed the form.

The week before we went to the center, Tracy and I began a "pre-oleation" diet—basically, we needed to suck down a lot of oil and clean out our digestive tracts in order to get the maximum effect from the detox. I tracked down ghee in a small grocery store; it is clarified butter sold by the jar. In solid form it's the color of honey and has the consistency of marzipan. Dal beans, the main ingredient in the rice-based *kitchari* recipe they sent me, were harder to find. I figured Indian takeout would do just fine; how much harm could a Samosa do?

Tracy phoned me on the Friday before we left. "So what's the deal with this ghee?" she asked. "I'm eating a couple slices at a time. How are you getting it down?"

"It's butter. I'm melting it. Taking it like medicine."

"Melting it—I never thought of that!" We both erupted into laughter, our pre-oleating stomachs cramping so hard. "This is gonna be *hilarious*," she cackled.

I barely slept the night before I traveled to New Mexico. And I never sleep on planes. So while flying the friendly skies, I listened to Madonna on my iPod (*Tell me everything I'm not, But please don't tell me to stop.  . . .*) and went through a stack of magazines I'd brought with me, tearing out the articles I wanted to keep. *Vogue, Vanity Fair, Us Weekly, Glamour, Self, The New Yorker.* I couldn't believe I was leaving all my media behind. Walking away from e-mails and phone calls from Oxygen for a week. My pen—my fave pen, a Uni-ball Roller—exploded on me on the plane, so I got ink all over my hands. They weren't quite henna tattoos.

I wrote in my journal (around the massive ink blobs):

*Fearful that I'll get in trouble. Fearful that they/I will find something out that's terrible about myself—that the Wegener's is my fault; I did something wrong. Scared to be touched, scared to take my body seriously, scared to give up any neurotic NYC Jewish OCD consumer stuff color noise smoke swear words dirt fat glass champagne Amex sushi carbs bitter jealous fuming sharp in exchange for peace blessing silence organic lady in leotard with hemp shopping bag.*

I flipped through the materials the center had sent me. They gave me a little background on what was apparently the world's oldest method of healing: "Ayurveda, the science of life, has brought true health and wellness to millions of individuals throughout the ages with simple changes in daily living practices. Incorporating just a few of these proven methods into your lifestyle can bring about radical changes in your life. This ancient art of healing has been practiced continuously for over five thousand years. The principles of many natural healing systems now familiar in the West, such as Homeopathy and Polarity Therapy, have their roots in Ayurveda. Ayurvedic practices restore the balance and harmony of the individual, resulting in self-healing, good health and longevity." I could use a giant shot of harmony.

When I arrived at the airport, Tracy was waiting for me at the gate with a big vinyl bag strapped to the front of her. It was all the luggage she brought. I had a huge rolling case and nine carry-ons. On the way out of the southwestern-style airport—all brown and turquoise—I tossed my pile of magazines into a trash bin. Bye-bye, Britney & *NSYNC. So long, supercouple splits: Tom & Nicole, Russell & Meg, J-Lo & Puffy ("Will she ever find love again?"). I'd also told my parents that they weren't going to hear from me for the entire week, which was unheard of. Pretty much like telling them that I was going deep undercover in 'Nam, and if they saw a car full of men in uniform coming up the driveway they'd know I was KIA. With the exception of promised phone reports to Sam, I wanted a full-throttle detox from Regular Life. I couldn't believe it. I'd never even been to a yoga class, and now I was in freakin' New Mexico about to get my insides turned out.

Albuquerque was a suburb like any other; only this one was planted in what looked like a giant crater. Desert. It was quiet at five-ish on a Sunday. We had no other directions, so we had a cabbie drop us off at the Ayurvedic Center. It looked like a Montessori school, located on a busy intersection. Across the way was a strip mall with a big supermarket and several AVAILABLE FOR RENT signs. I was secretly grateful to see the supermarket, because I knew I wouldn't be able to make it the whole week without sneaking some real, horrible, processed, trans-fat-alicious food.

Even Quaker Instant Oatmeal—Cinnamon & Spice, of course—would do it for me.

No one was at the center when we arrived by cab, but a handsome guy drove up in a Jeep. "Hey, my name's Mack. I work at the center. Where are you staying?"

"Uh, Lotus House?"

"That's real close, but too far to drag your suitcases. How 'bout I take you over there?" This would be a major no-no in New York, but perfectly friendly in New Mexico. Mack helped us sling our stuff up in the Jeep, one of those safari-looking ones. It was the first time I'd ridden in a car that didn't have doors.

Thankfully, Lotus House looked pretty normal: a suburban house with a second story added on. The keys were in an envelope taped to the door, as Ray the owner had said they would be. When I walked in, I smelled incense. It was pretty warm in there. There was a little bench in the foyer and shoes under it. I guessed you weren't supposed to wear shoes inside. Moving in, I saw French doors with lacy curtains, and beyond the curtains some of those Indian paintings with gold flakes on them. There was someone behind the curtain. There always is.

The bathrooms were clean, but strangely, there were little plastic hooks adhered to the wall about two feet off the ground, which was a little low for a towel rack. The bedrooms were spare but neat, with towels stacked in the closets. A complete list of directions and rules was posted in the closet. It mentioned using "a different kind of towel for the enemas." Like it was an assumed thing. Nerve-racking.

The kitchen was pretty empty except for lots of pots and

strainers. (What the heck was gonna need straining at a spa? I thought.) The shelves were lined with books about Ayurveda, Jyotish (Indian astrology), alternative healing, carpentry . . . and another little altar area was packed inside the fireplace. The mystery man finally came out of the curtained room. He was about our age (twenty-six, actually). Cute, with curly hair, Buddy Holly glasses, a black turtleneck, his hands stuffed in pockets and his pants slung low on his hips. His name was Ryan. When Tracy asked him where he lived, he curtly replied, "I'm a nomad, but right now I live with my mother."

Ray came home. He had short shaved hair and a long, white-streaked, wiry beard. He told us that he practiced alternative medicine and used to work at the center but quit because they didn't pay enough. He'd built the additions on to Lotus House himself. "Did you grow up in New Mexico?" I asked.

"Naw," he said. "A little town in Michigan. You never heard of it."

"Try me," I said.

"It's near a place called Keego Harbor. Not a town, actually, more of a township. Bloomfield Hills." That's where I grew up. Who needed an enema? I nearly took a dump in my pants.

"Where did you go to high school?" I asked, knowing already that he'd say the same school as me. Yup—he was Bloomfield Hills Andover High School, class of '74. I was class of '89. Ray's family still lived two blocks away from my parents. I accepted that something supernatural was going to happen on our trip.

I suggested to Tracy that we head back to the center. The orientation meeting wasn't for another fifteen minutes, and it was only a five-minute walk through a soccer field and park, but I didn't want to rush and sweat. A few people were milling around when we arrived. In the article, the lady had written about all the new best friends she'd made at the center, but this was a motley crew: an Indian guy in white robes, another in Western dress. A very thin, white woman in sweatpants. A sparkly woman with a British accent. A white woman with curly hair and glasses and a milky complexion offered to tell me all about her guru. (Later that week she slipped me a CD of that guru's teachings to take back to New York and said, "Listen. I think you'll get a lot out of this." But I lost the CD.) Tracy and I stood out as newbies, looking at each other nervously. Finally Ryan joined us.

A man I assumed was one of the center's directors walked in the front door. "I'm Bob," he said. I didn't know you could work at an Ayurvedic Center and have a "Hey, buddy!" name like Bob. He was maybe in his mid-forties. Bob had a mustache and a discoloration on his nose that made me nervous. He wore a Members Only–style jacket that had the words VALE TINO sewn on the pocket. Not Valentino; Vale Tino. Obviously not a materialistic dude. Might be played by William H. Macy in the movie. When he unlocked the door and flicked on the fluorescent lights, I was hit with a waft of indistinct Indian spices and incense. The smell was a turn-off and a temptation at the same time (kind of like picking at belly lint). We crammed into a little lobby space with mismatched chairs. There was a table on wheels with hot food plates on it, some jars filled with limes and crushed garlic, with parsley-looking something, too. Chinese-food cartons sat on the bottom shelf, next to plastic silverware. A hot drink canister read

AGNI. I noticed a water tank with cold water in the corner. I was so relieved to drink it, but the cups were those little tiny ones they have at the dentist's office and I could only lap a couple of sips at a time. I felt total compassion for thirsty dogs.

"Feel free to eat some *kitchari*," Bob directed. Oh, that's the thing I was supposed to cook (but didn't) during pre-oleation. I ate mung dal delivered from an Indian restaurant instead. I'd assumed it was pronounced "kitsch-AH-ree." Did he say "KITCH-a-dee"? People started serving themselves from the hot pans as if they knew what they were doing. "You can have as much as you like, but don't eat if you're full," ordered Bob. I scooped some of the yellow soupy stuff into a bowl. It was hot temperature-wise; I expected it to taste like curry but it didn't. Bland. There were some spices and rock salt to put in it, but I couldn't trust that stuff. I was definitely going to have to hit that grocery store.

Bob told us that he wanted to give us a little talk "about cause and effect and the like," but he would show us around the facilities first. I had a major headache that I assumed was from lack of sleep and dehydration and general mind melt. Turns out Tracy's head was aching, too, as was Ryan's, our housemate. They both looked uncomfortable during the tour. I was depending on Tracy to be my rock. If she burned out, then I was gonna lose it. Bob pointed out a meditation room that we were free to use anytime (thanks but no thanks), and the suites where we'd have our actual detoxing treatments. We sat back down in the lobby and Bob solicited questions. The Indian guy in the Western clothes asked if we could go to movies during the week, a suggestion that was treated with somewhat haughty dismissal. I asked, "Bob, how can we work out any emotional conflicts like, uh, resistance, for example, that we might feel during the week?"

"Try silence," he said.

Tracy and Ryan both opted to return to Lotus House to crash with their bad headaches. I didn't want to miss any important info, so I stayed for the Talk.

The Talk was frustrating. Bob had an unusual speech pattern; he'd speak a full sentence, then say, "So . . . ," then pause, then start up again. "Let's talk a little bit about cause and effect. (Pause). So . . ." He didn't seem to be too big on eye contact. Actually, besides Ray, he might have been the least demonstrative guy I'd ever met. I needed a little more encouragement here.

Bob gave us more on the Ayurvedic basics. The theory was that everyone is born with a unique constitution, or *dosha*, made of three mind/body types: *vata* (ether and air), *pitta* (fire and water), and *kapha* (water and earth). *Vata* controlled breathing and movement/fear and anxiety, *pitta* represented digestion and metabolism/anger and jealousy, and *kapha* was all about lubrication and immunity/attachment and greed (Madonna says she's a *pitta/vata*). The theory, as I understood it, was that from the moment we were born, this constitution was thrown out of whack by poor digestion, pollution, and negative emotions, leaving us with our current imbalance, or *vikruti*. The goal was to get our *vikruti* back to match our *prakruti* (*dosha* combo at birth) so we could ideally be disease-free. Bob talked about balance and past lives and the toxicity of negative emotion. His take on cause and effect was similar to that of Buddhism (and Kabbalah, for that matter). It was overwhelming, confusing, and the only thing I could really grasp was his suggestion that I had caused my own disease by having human emotions and living on the verge of the twenty-first century. Too much for me to handle right off the bat. Plus they rolled away that kitsch-a-ree/kitch-a-dee cart before I'd really gotten enough to eat, so I was screwed. Again, Bob recommended silence during PK treatments. He told us not to bring bags, jewelry, money, watches, etc. They wanted us in bed by 10 p.m., up at dawn. My head was pounding. By the time I got out of there I desperately needed fresh air. I couldn't figure out how I was going to do this for a week. This was worse than summer camp; and this time I hadn't even been forced—I'd chosen to go! That Sunday night, the big Albuquerque sky was overcast. I couldn't even get simple inspiration from seeing stars that were invisible in the skies of New York.

Everyone was asleep when I arrived back at Lotus, so I couldn't debrief Tracy. I'd secretly hoped to convince her that we should take our yet un-enemaed towels and run for it, but no luck. It was only about about 9 p.m. I tried to stretch time by meticulously unpacking my stuff and putting my room in order. I poked around, trying to find cold water, but there wasn't any. So I read a book from Ray's library about building dormers, twiddled my thumbs, and eventually fell asleep.

At 6 a.m. the following morning, I met with Bob. He was going to be my PK coordinator for the week. It was warm in the center's lobby, and I was still thirsting for my fill of cold water. I also couldn't stop sweating. I needed information, clarification, and hydration, not necessarily in that order.

The lobby had fake wood paneling and a cheap Styrofoam ceiling with all the little holes in it. I felt like I was waiting to interview with a temp agency. My nerves were already frayed and I hadn't even been in Albuquerque for twenty-four hours. I was wearing my workout uniform, stretch pants, and a plus-size Danskin T-shirt over an exercise bra. I didn't have my watch or my cell phone, and so felt completely untethered. My comfort zone was approximately eighteen hundred miles away in a city packed with tall pointy buildings and a Korean nail salon on every corner. *What am I doing here?* I asked my rational self. I looked down on a side table and curiously found a memo titled "What You Are Doing Here." It was packed with Sanskrit words that I still couldn't understand. I picked up an old well-handled copy of *Yoga Journal* and looked at the smiling, moon-eyed model on the cover. *If they're trying to show you that yoga is for everyone, why are the people on the covers always photographed in such intricate poses? I'm not a pretzel. Why should I bother to give this stuff a chance?* I charged my rational mind, just as I glanced down at a page of the magazine titled something like, "Why You Should Bother to Give This Stuff a Chance." Gulp.

Bob stepped out of his tiny office and called me in. "So . . . ," he began, taking notes and avoiding eye contact. This guy and I were not on the same page. I tried to explain Wegener's to Bob, but he seemed much more focused on the food I ate (mucho carbs and sweets, thanks to prednisone) and what time I went to bed (never). He wanted to see my tongue. *Blaaah.* I made the mistake of telling Bob that I hadn't had a natural bowel movement since the early 1990s, so he thought that an enema was in order. He handed me a big scary plastic bag and tube contraption that I was supposed to use posttreatment that afternoon. How? It wasn't like I could Google up "how to give yourself an enema" in the meditation room. Before I could get a handle on anything, Bob said it was time to meet with Dr. Rai and he'd explain it all later.

He walked me to another wing of the center, which was even warmer.

We passed by some sort of gift shop—*shopping, thank Ganesh!*\*— and went down a flight of stairs into a carpeted yoga studio. I recognized the infamous Dr. Rai from his photo in the magazine article. He was perched in a folding chair in front of several rows of students. They were his graduate students, and like his patients they came from around the world to study with him. There was a table with doctor's office paper spread on it, and an empty chair at the far end of it. I had to slip off my shoes again (I'd packed lace-up sneakers—why hadn't they told me to bring slip-ons?) and sat in the chair. I'd imagined doctors on rounds with residents in white coats, but these class members (men, women, young, old, Indian, Caucasian) looked like summer camp reunionees. They were very smiley. No shoes. No desks or tables, just open binders

---

\* Ganesh is my favorite of the Hindu dieties—the elephant-faced figure known as the Remover of Obstacles.

on their laps so they could take notes. This could be the dawning of the Age of Aquarius.

Dr. Rai was slender, with smooth brown skin and a warm smile. He had an air of gentle elegance. He wore wire-rimmed glasses. I felt like I'd seen that profile somewhere . . . ah, yes. He looked like Smithers from *The Simpsons*, only Indian. He wore several jeweled rings on his hand and, like Bob, he didn't make much eye contact. When he finally looked at me, I felt as though he had seen my type a million times before but would kindly indulge a nonbeliever once again. He flipped through the notes that Bob had given him, and then gave the floor to me. "Shan-kar," he said in his Indian accent, a wink in his voice. "Tell us why you're here."

I explained my Wegener's diagnosis, with Bob adding in salient details whenever I paused. I also acknowledged my weight, telling them that I ate what I thought of as a balanced diet, though they'd probably disagree. This fostered a laugh from the class. Dr. Rai asked what I did for a living, and I told him I worked in television. "Oh," he said to the students, "then we know she lives in the fifth chakra." They all laughed. I was like, *What chou talkin' bout, Willis? Take your little chakra joke and stuff it in my enema bag.*

Dr. Rai directed me to sit on the table so he could take my pulse. I expected him to grip one wrist and stare at his watch with the other, as doctors always had. To my surprise, he clasped each of my wrists with three fingers, and began to . . . play them, almost like flutes. He shut his eyes and listened attentively, murmuring to himself. The class sat silently. I didn't realize at the time that he was meditating.

He asked me, "You had pneumonia when you were twelve, thirteen or so?"

"Twelve," I said. Hmm, I didn't remember listing that on my forms.

"You had surgery on your nose?" he inquired.

"Yes, a biopsy."

He clicked his tongue. "Why do they have to cut into you? Into people?" He sighed. "It is your brother who has asthma?" Yeah, it was. But what did Josh have to do with this? And how did Rai know about *his* medical history? Maybe he had psychic insight.

Rai asked me to lie down on the table while he examined my tongue and my eyes. I wasn't sure whether I should look at him or straight up at the ceiling, so I switched back and forth. He touched different, tender joints on my body. Then, when he pressed his palm on my stomach, it really hurt, and not just because I was pretty bloated. When he tapped my sinuses I flinched—maybe a bit too much, like a basketball player tumbling for a foul, but he didn't seem as dismayed by the Wegener's symptoms as I'd expected he'd be.

Finally he nodded his head and turned to speak to the class in a tone that was both analytical and respectful, using those terms *dosha, prakruti* and *vikruti, kapha, pitta,* and *agni.* He stroked my arm. "Her skin, this is *shlakshna.*" *Slakshna* skin—whatever it was, that seemed to please him. He warned the students that they might have trouble reading my pulse due to my "adipose tissue"—a delicate way of saying that I was too fat. At least he was delicate.

When he invited the class members to take my pulse, they formed two lines and each held a wrist, making eye contact and smiling before they checked it. Each one gave me a supportive squeeze before letting go of my wrist. No doctor had ever done that. I sat back down in the chair as Dr. Rai began to deliver my diagnosis. They scribbled it down.

"*Prakruti,*" he said. "*Vata* two, *pitta* three, *kapha* one. *Vikruti . . . vata* two, *pitta* three-point-five, and *kapha . . .* I almost say four." This drew a gasp from the class. In his estimation, I had too much *pitta* (fire) and waaay too much *kapha* (sludge). "But let's try *kapha* three-point-five, *pitta* pushing *kapha.*" That meant my fire overload was throwing my *kapha* so out of whack. If I could get a grip on the *pitta* by detoxing, the *kapha* would follow. Rai read off a litany of Sanskrit instructions, checking them off on his sheet. He prescribed different oils and herbs, and something called chromatherapy. "The most important thing," he explained, "is to get the *agni* going. We must get her *agni* burning." *Agni* was inner digestive fire. Chronic constipation was doing me no favors.

Here's what was extra creepy: This Ayurveda theory kind of made sense to me. I wasn't Indian, but I had an Indian-sounding name (Shanker, Shankar, so close). But the stuff about the fire, and the constitution, Rai knowing about my pneumonia . . . What if he was right? What if Turner & Company were only making me sicker, and this completely out-there process would make me well? As resistant as I was to the concept of "emotional" illness, and wary of healers like Rai, it occurred to me, Maybe he's the guy. Perhaps my problem required tools a Western doctor didn't have in his medicine bag. One med does not fit all. Like losing weight or finding Mr. Right, there was no Easy-Bake Oven when it came to health. I always hated the way doctors spoke about a "magic bullet" for weight loss, as if you could just shoot the fat person and she'd deflate like a balloon. A pill wasn't a cure-all, either. During Rai's examination, I felt hope stirring. We couldn't have had less in common, but still I wondered if somehow this ageless Indian intuitive medicine man—a guy who prescribed leeches, for crying out loud—knew something that the white coats didn't. Maybe he was the guru who could take Wendy Dumpty and put her back together again.

That afternoon I met my PK technicians, Luscha and Sandra. Luscha was tall, thin, and German with blond hair in braided pigtails. Sandra was rounder and shorter, with a brown bob and a warm smile. Both wore white nursing uniforms. They ushered me into the *abhyanga* massage room I'd seen the night before, where a synchronized oil massage was supposed to move toxins out of my muscles and into my digestive tract so they could be disposed of. Little elephants dangled from the ceiling, and big plastic jars of oil were stacked everywhere. Ghee central. In that small room, as in every center room, a miniature rock water fountain gurgled. A large massage table lined with plastic and covered with white bedsheets took up most of the space. I peeled off my workout clothes and hung them on hooks, then scuffled under the top sheet totally naked. I glanced through the large window behind me. It seemed incongruous to see a midnight blue Dodge Neon in the parking lot upside down through the blinds when I was about to be metaphysically transformed.

The girls knocked on the door and entered. "Are you warm enough?" asked Sandra in a gentle voice. Warm enough? They had no idea. Apparently my ongoing self-induced sweatshop was part of my *pitta* imbalance, and when I was all better I'd be cool as a cuke. "Would you prefer music or silence?" I opted for silence as Bob had suggested. I didn't know if I should watch them, or keep my eyes open or closed, so I did a mish-mosh as they prepared bottles of oil and jars of herbs. Finally each of them stood on a side of me and laid a hand on my hands. "We're going to start by chanting," said Luscha. "You are welcome to join us if you want."

Oh shit, I thought. I'm Jewish. Are we even allowed to chant?* Luscha and Sandra made eye contact with each other. Then Luscha closed her eyes, while Sandra left hers open and turned away.

"*Haaaa Rheeee Oooohm. Haaaa Rheeee Oooohm . . .*"

It was a beautiful sound, but I was glad it was over quickly since it was potentially sacrilegious. I tried to breathe, close my eyes, and relax. Luscha began by pouring warm oil over my scalp and massaging it in. Sandra was down by my feet. They worked silently and in tandem, and I could feel an occasional warm pour

---

* According to traditional Jewish law, no. You're invoking another religion's dieties.

of more oil. Luscha asked me to tip my head back and put some sort of drops in my nostrils. This was called *nasya*, and it was powerful enough to make me cough. I tasted sesame oil and licorice, ghee and some unrecognizable spice in the back of my throat. I worried that the nose drops would make my sinuses more congested, but why had I come all this way if I wasn't going to at least try them? Still, I asked them not to pour oil in my ears since I had an infection in my nasopharynx. After a while, they moved down to my feet and began to work their way up my legs, in tandem. Long, smooth strokes on my legs, my arms, my stomach and chest. When they poured oil down the back of my neck, it flowed down to my armpits and felt strangely exhilarating. Half an hour later, they lifted the top sheet and asked me to turn over. I opened my eyes and was surprised to see the sheets covered in yellow oil and strands of my hair—I realized the girls must have been picking hair off me the whole time. It was difficult to turn over; I felt epically tired. My boobs were in the way so I had to do some manual shifting, and then I fit my face into one of those massage face-space thingies. They worked on my legs, arms, and shoulders. They poured oil down my back, and it flowed into my ass crack and dripped into my vulva (an unsettling but surprisingly pleasant sensation). My mind raced. I mulled over my friends, my work, my disease. It was hard to let go and relax.

Almost an hour passed by the time they finished. One of them put a hand on my exposed palm, and the other on the small of my back. They placed their opposite hands on my back and feet. It felt like they were forming triangles, or hearts. They asked me to turn over again and began to chant once more, each holding a hand. Sandra gave me a squeeze and a smile as they quietly walked out of the room.

I was utterly exhausted and more than relaxed; I could hardly move. They'd treated me as delicately as a baby, or an Indian princess. Those women had healing hands. I felt like Dorothy and her pals when they got the curly-twirly makeover in the Emerald City. Maybe "Rub rub here, rub rub there, and a couple of tra-la-las . . ." was the Oz-ian version of "I Ia Rhee Oooohm." I still had to go to the *swedana* room for individualized herbal sweat therapy (as a *pitta* person, I hated steam; Tracy, as a *vata* girl, relished it), then shift into *shirodhara*, a half-hour pour of warm oil directly on my forehead which was rumored to stimulate out-of-body experiences. Turner would flip if he could see all this. I felt very peaceful. For the first time since I'd arrived, I felt relieved that I was going to do *panchakarma* five days in row.

# 5

# Deeper & Deeper

believe that women have two subjects we could talk about until the day we die and still not say enough: weight and waste. Fat and shit. I rarely meet a woman unwilling to share her entire weight loss saga with me. And it's not like I have to provoke someone into revealing that she's constipated, has irritable bowel syndrome, or craps eleven times a day. Sometimes I think I'm a kind of crap magnet, an emotional toilet for everyone else's digestive drama. Maybe it's because I give off a maternal vibe, so somehow women feel safe confessing to me (I am the Protector, after all). I understand the anatomical self-interest completely, and I know it's a symbolic Freudian thing. Madonna once said she's had her most contemplative moments while she's sitting on the crapper. I'm fascinated by number two, too. For a while I wrote a blog called dailydoody.com, in which I'd recount my daily evacuations. It wasn't so much my yearning to express the details of my digestion as a bet that I could write an idiotic blog about anything and someone would read it. I was "The Dooder"; Sam's sign-on was "Just Pooping By." I found a pair of Swedish stuffed animals named Pee (who looked like a big yellow teardrop) and Poo (who looked like a big brown fluffy squirt) and made them my website icons.

Swedes are hilarious.

Anyway, with all the crazy stuff that I've experienced in the name of health, the one that everyone is the most curious about is colonics. I've tried three types: the little squeeze bottles that you buy at the drugstore, the big bags and tubes that they gave me at the Ayurvedic Center, and the full-on, strap-me-into-the-machine, you-do-the-dirty-work professional colonic. There are several reasons why people get them, including detoxification of the digestive tract, relief for acute constipation, prepping for medical exams, and becoming a Hollywood star. The real question is why someone would administer them, considering that a colonic is usually considered a medical no-no and has a gross factor of $n$ to the nth degree. Money is a motivator, but in my experience the main reason anyone gives healing treatments for a living—colonics, massages, acupuncture—is that they are converts themselves. They were sick, someone suggested they do this wacky thing, and it worked. I've gone for professional colonics in New York City three times, and each time the technicians were delighted to do it. They weren't freaked out because they knew something that I, as a new patient, didn't: There would be no explosion. I would not lose bowel control and spray like one of those Crazy Daisy lawn sprinklers that kids play in. Yes, there was a feeling of fullness. There was a moment when I said to myself, "Oh, dear, I don't think this is gonna work." But I breathed through it, and it actually felt kind of enjoyable, and I could even kibitz with the technician while I was getting cleaned out. Afterward, they tried to upsell me on a nine-week regimen, threatening that even the littlest bit of Hostess/Splenda/can-of-Coke-that-could-rot-a-copper-penny* would destroy my newly cleaned colon from the inside out, but I demurred.

In March 2001, in the bathroom of the Lotus House in Albuquerque, New Mexico, I didn't yet know all that. I opened the big paper bag Bob had given me that morning. It was the kind that my mom packed lunches in, but no PB&J was to be found. Inside was an enema kit called a *basti*. It included a sturdy medical plastic bag with ounce measurements notched on it; a long thin hose that had curled around itself; a bottle of yellow sesame oil; and two plastic bags of what looked like the kind of weed a senior would sell a naïve freshman, aka dirt from the shrubs outside the garage. The herbs had been ground especially for me as dictated by Dr. Rai's prescription. They didn't look like they should go into my body, especially if my rectum was the entry point. These were exit-only herbs.

Rai was convinced that digestion, more than any of the massage, meditation, or treatments, was the key to improving my health. "Turn up the *agni*, the digestive fire," he'd said. That was the reason we only ate *kitchari*; it was easy to digest so our colons could focus on bigger projects. For me, it was *basti* or bust. Rai didn't believe that I had an autoimmune problem; he thought

---

* Not true, BTW—a can of Coke cannot dissolve pennies, nails, or rust stains. A glass of orange juice contains more citric acid than a can of Coke. Not that you should be sucking down all that high-fructose corn syrup. If you're going to drink "the Real Thing," look for the real thing, Coke made with sugar.

poor digestion that led to body toxicity was causing the Wegener's symptoms. I assumed with all that fire shooting around my system my digestion would be zooming along, but apparently my *kapha* factor was slowing everything down. The excess *pitta* was responsible for my overheating and my temper. Tracy was fine on *pitta* and *kapha*, but her *vata* was completely out of whack, explaining why she was always cold and prone to headaches. Ryan chose not to explain his imbalance to us.

I finally discovered the purpose for all those strainers stocked in the Lotus House kitchen: *basti* prep. I had to boil up my herbs, strain them, add them to the simmering oil, pour the whole concoction into the *basti* bag, then somehow get it up in me at an hour of day predesignated by Dr. Rai. (A warning to the uninitiated: This process takes time. You do *not* want to rush when you are going to shoot hot, herb-enhanced oil up your butt. It must cool down. Some of my fellow PK detoxers learned this lesson the hard way.) Once the solution had cooled to room temperature, I funneled a few cups' worth into the bag. It swelled a little bigger than the inflatable water wings a kid wears for safety in a swimming pool. I went into the bathroom that I shared with Tracy and locked the door.

The clinicians at the center used to administer *basti*s to PK clients, but it was declared illegal around the same time they had to discontinue bloodletting and forced purgation. I took a set of *basti* towels from the closet and spread one out on the bathroom floor. I placed a few paper towels on top of that. At the sink, I poked one end of the tube into the *basti* bag and took the cap off the other end. Bob had recommended we put a little oil on the tip before inserting it. (I can't believe Bob was the guy who explained this whole thing to me. It was like having the "Bueller, Bueller" teacher explain where babies come from.) Time for a test run in the sink. As I raised the bag, the fluid rushed through the tube and came out the open end. To stop the flow, I needed to lower the bag below the other end of the tube. It was a very simple gravity issue, but regrettably I hadn't been paying attention in fourth grade, when I should have figured this stuff out. I recapped the open end and hung the *basti* bag on one of those little plastic hooks on the wall (so that's what those suckers were for!). I lay down on the towel on my left side, curled into a fetal position, uncapped the tube, and ever so gently placed it where it needed to go.

Stretching my arm above my head, I lifted the bag off of the hook and . . . *whoosh*. Whoa, whoa! Nothing messy, but just way too fast. I lowered the bag and the flow stopped. Okay, okay. Not a terrible sensation, kind of warm but very strange, because I was going in through the out door. Slower this time, I lifted the bag from the hook. Once I realized that everything was going to be sanitary and controlled, I let a third of the liquid in the bag drain into me as I'd been instructed, then replaced the bag on the hook, recapped the tube, and turned over on my back. I was supposed to wait for five minutes and then do another third of liquid lying on my left side, wait another five, and do the final third on my right.

What does one think about when one is on one's back in a bathroom with a tube up her butt in New Mexico? I tried to focus on breathing, especially when I began to feel a cramp, and then gained a little more confidence as I got through it. I thought about Ben Affleck, because I'd read somewhere that he had done colonics, and then I thought about Gwyneth because she seemed like the type who would do this kind of thing on a regular basis. Then I remembered that I was trying not to think about media but about my cells and my spirit, so I breathed again. I mused about my little brother Joshie getting that dime stuck up his nose, and then I deliberated about kids swallowing loose change and bubble gum, and then I remembered a special I'd seen on the Discovery Channel called *The 101 Most Unusual Things Ever Found in the Human Body*. The list included jelly jars, silverware, and a section of a ski pole that had gone in a guy's head on one side and came out the other without damaging his brain. The *most* unusual thing was found in an Indian man who had a sixty-pound tumor in his stomach. When surgeons finally operated and sliced the tumor open, they found fifty-nine pounds of goo and a calcified twin that the guy had ingested while gestating in his mother's uterus. That was worth waiting for.

I doubted I'd find a calcified twin in my colon, but I did recall an urban myth about some lady disgorging a Barbie shoe that she had swallowed when she was a little girl. I pictured it as a teeny rubber pink high-heeled mule that the Mattel folks had paired with an age-inappropriate Barbie negligee. The chances were slim that I'd discover that level of treasure, but I have to admit I was hoping at the very least to unearth one of those little toys in the plastic eggs you can buy for twenty-five cents out of a gumball machine.

After fifteen minutes, when I'd taken in most of the *basti* and had turned my body on all three sides (like gyro meat on a spit at

Olga's Kitchen at the food court in a suburban Detroit shopping mall) to let it move around inside my colon, I *delicately* went for the dismount. I had to get up off the floor while maintaining my composure, and with muscles tight and breath firm, move over and sit on the toilet for the final release. Which I did. Like a Buddha perched on porcelain, I turned my focus inward and let go. There it was again: letting go. But nothing happened.

Impossible. Maybe I was still clenching somewhere? I had just soaked up a giant bag of warm, dirty oil. There was no way it could have escaped without my knowledge. I recomposed myself, released again, and still nothing happened.

Bob hadn't mentioned this as a possible outcome. Had I strained the oil well enough? Maybe one of those little twigs had jammed up the works somewhere. I'd imagined it like *Last of the Mohicans*, where one little chunk of herb could leap like a tiny Daniel Day-Lewis into a rushing waterfall, but it would still all flow out. But it didn't. By this time I'd been in the bathroom for over an hour. Tracy needed to get in there, and I needed to run to my *abhyanga* massage appointment with Sandra and Luscha. So I got up, put away my towels, gently donned my workout clothes, and hustled over to the center.

When I told Bob what hadn't happened, I believe he was almost impressed. He assumed that my bowels were so dry that they had absorbed the entire *basti*. That was why my system was on shutdown—so much *pitta* that my digestive system had stopped functioning. This *basti* would amp up the *agni*, which would remove the toxic *ama* and make me a happy, healthy person. Secretly I hoped my mean, dry season would get Dr. Rai's attention. Then I wouldn't be one of the by-the-number seekers; I would certainly be one of the most remarkable patients he'd ever had. I could imagine his locker room chat with Dr. Oz and Andrew Weil: "Oh, Mehmet, Andy, did I ever tell you about the time I had Shan-kar and she did the *basti* five times and nothing came out?"

Every day I did the same routine: Wake up a 6 a.m., do my *basti* with disappointing results. I'd head over to the center for my *abhyanga* massage, while Tracy and Ryan stayed back at Lotus House, their treatment schedules the opposite of mine. I suffered through a few overheated minutes of sweating in the *swedana* (Miss *Pitta* hated sweating!), then blissed out in total relaxation during the *shirodhara*. When the pour was over, they'd dust my body with ground sandalwood and chickpea powder, making me smell like a tantalizing Indian appetizer. I'd take a long shower to rinse off the dust and unsuccessfully try to wring the pungent oil out of my hair. I'd join Tracy in the lobby where we'd eat *kitchari*, less and less each day as our hunger faded, our skin cleared, and our eyes grew bright. In the afternoons I'd rest or try restorative yoga. I wasn't that familiar with yoga, but we'd basically just lie propped up in stretchy positions on our mats for a few minutes at a time. No wonder everyone loved this stuff; it was exercise you could sleep through! At night the PK clients were invited to attend Dr. Rai's graduate classes, which started with chanting and ended with a drum circle. By 8:30 or 9 p.m. we were wiped out. Tracy and I would chill in the meditation room at Lotus House, with Ryan quietly dangling nearby on a couch. (Ryan was brilliant at the *basti*. We called him "the *Basti* King" and I think he was quite proud.) We burned sticks of incense while he listened to us trade stories and debate Big Questions about creativity, feminism, and relationships, his eyes fixed on Tracy.

Wait a second: had PK love blossomed between Ryan and Tracy at the Lotus House while I was away? Maybe they were both drinking the *kapha* Kool-Aid, sharing one tall icy glass with two straws. I got pissed. I was all *pitta*, all the time. Why was Ryan attracted to Tracy but not me? I wanted the attention. I was the sick one. The more I learned about my crazy, overfiery constitution the angrier I got: What am I doing here? Why is this illness a part of my life? What if I die? What if I don't? There were twelve thousand things I had to change (food combinations, waking and sleeping time, meditation, tongue scraping, herbs, oils, teas, visualization) to upgrade my karma and make myself well. The one thing I couldn't do—the most important of all—was the *basti*. Clearly I was either unable or unwilling to let go.

# 6

# Open Your Heart

When I go to a healer who seems to be connected to the universe in a way that I'm not, my brain argues back and forth about all the yogis and meditators and believers: They must know something that I don't. But, my rational brain argues back, if they're really right, then why don't we simply do what they tell us to do and get better? Then I remember that the word *doctor* comes from the Latin for "teacher."

Halfway through the week of PK, Bob offered me a deal. Part of Dr. Rai's analysis could include a reading of our astrological charts. It wasn't the same as a Western Zodiac chart—even though I knew mine was also heavy on the fire signs. The chart was in Jyotish, the Vedic astrological system. It looked like a tic-tac-toe chart with little stars and dots in each of the windows. Along with the reading, Bob said we could write down a couple of questions he would give to Rai, who would derive the answers from our charts. "Careful what you ask," Bob warned. "Don't ask a question if you're not ready to hear the answer."

Here I was with an amazing one-time limited offer from Dr. Rai: He could tell me my future. I jotted down:

*Am I going to live a long life?*

*Am I going to have children?*

*Am I following the right spiritual path?*

Looking back, I wish I'd been a bit more specific. The next day at our consultation, Bob returned with the answers. "So . . . I spoke with Dr. Rai. You asked, 'Am I going to live a long life?' Well, you're going to live a good life."

"But a 'good' life isn't the same as a 'long' life," I clarified.

"I told you not to ask if you weren't ready to hear the answer."

Okey-doke. I moved on to the next one. "What about children?"

"There are children on your chart, but there's a problem there. It's like you're separated from children somehow."

That was two strikes.

"But don't worry," Bob assured me. "Rai says you are definitely following the right spiritual path."

Who cares about my spiritual path! That one was a throw-away; I only asked it to impress Rai. I was destined for a short, childless future? How awful! Then again, according to Rai's belief system, I was going to get reincarnated anyway. I'd be able to try again in my next life.

On our final day, Tracy and I were scheduled for chroma-therapy, which were color healing sessions. I physically was walking on sunshine by that point—my system as clean as it had been since before I started trick-or-treating, even without a successful *basti*. Tracy and I had also cried a lot of toxic energy out of systems during our nightly chats. While the detox was clearly a step in the right direction, I still felt disappointed not to be a standout case for the staff or Dr. Rai himself. PK had been revealing, and rewarding, but nothing had zipped *kundalini*-style down from the collective unconscious and opened up my brain. I had yet to undergo a transformative experience, when past lives would jump up before me and explain everything, as the PK brochure promised.

Tracy left for her chromatherapy appointment while I packed up my stuff. When I arrived in the treatment suite, Tracy came out of the chromatherapy room. As she walked toward me, her face was gray. "Trace . . . are you okay?" I asked. She pulled me close and then waved me off, muttering, "I can't talk about it." She hurried into the center's meditation room and shut the door.

Now I was supposed to go in *there*, after it freaked out someone as experienced as Tracy? Oh my God, what the hell was "color therapy" anyway? What were they going to do to me? What if it was like that Scrooge thing, and they'd show me a horrible vision of my short, unchilded, good-spiritual-path-following life? Even worse, what if they could look into my soul and truly see what was wrong with me? I wasn't sure I wanted to know.

I entered a *shirodhara* treatment room, but instead of a pot of simmering oil above my head, I saw a vertical row of lights, a rig like you'd see on a community theater stage. There were seven lights, corresponding with each of the seven chakras, covered with colored gels: from the bottom, red, yellow, orange, green, blue, purple, and white. I was going to take a trip under the rainbow.

I like anything organized, especially if it has rainbow colors. All that Roy G. Biv that I could draw with a box of Crayolas as a kid . . . yum yum. That's why I loved the chakra theory. The idea was that the body had seven different energy centers starting at the base of the spine and running up and out of the body, envisioned as wheels. Each chakra was associated with a different body part, a different system. It was like the Zodiac with five signs less to remember and in a straight line.

I peeled off my clothes just as I did for the *abhyanga*, clambered up on the table, and spread a towel over my body. Barbara, the technician, came in the room and smiled. Like Sandra and Luscha, she offered a loving vibe. "Why don't you start by taking a few deep breaths?" she asked. I could smell that oily Ayurveda scent, but my brain was already starting to move on to airports and transportation. She continued, "If you have any spirit guides you can call on, now would be a good time to do it." I scoffed. Yeah, I left my spirit guides in San Francisco, babe. Rack up your little lights and let's get the show on the road. I could not figure out what on earth had upset Tracy so badly.

Barbara laid a cool cloth over my eyes. I could hear paper rustling as she moved around the table. She began, "Dr. Rai prescribed a red light for the second chakra, skipping the first, or root chakra." The man prescribed lights? Why was I skipping one? Was I rootless? Was I special? Would I miss something that every-

one else was getting? I could sense Barbara down by my feet, zap-
ping me like I had static cling. "What are you doing to my toes?"
I asked.

"I'm not at your feet," she said. "I'm at your head. I just turned
on the red light." Zip-zip-zip-tingle. I assumed my feet had fallen
asleep because I heard a light switch click off at exactly the same
moment the tingling stopped. "Now I'm going to shine the yellow
light on your third chakra, which is just under your belly button.
This is the zone that affects the endocrine system and speeds up
digestion."

The tingling in my toes began again, and the sensation started
to whiz around my body, like a pinball tracking over my legs,
across my stomach, up my arm, across my chest, down the other
arm. I got really warm and broke into a sweat. "I'm feeling kind
of . . . zippy," I told her. I opened my eyes under the cloth and
tilted them down to get a sneak peek of what Barbara was doing
to me. Nothing. I had a towel over my hips, another one over my
breasts, and a yellow light shining just above my belly button.
Like a UFO about to land on the open field of my torso.

The light flipped off and the electricity stopped. I was panting
and starting to seriously perspire. How could I allow a Christmas
light to charge me up like this? Was I really that susceptible, or
longing for something major to happen so badly that a sixty-watt
bulb could do the trick? Barbara folded the towel up above my
waist, and then down over my stomach, so my chest and breasts
were exposed. "Is this okay with you?" she asked.

"Yeah, just give me a minute here." Shiz, Shanker, get your
wits together. You must need simple carbs in a bad way. Yes, I did

sneak into the grocery store earlier that week. I didn't buy anything; I just took a big whiff in the cereal aisle and walked back out the door. "Okay, you can move on," I said assuredly.

She flipped another switch. "This is the green light on the fourth chakra, the heart chakra. It is connected to love and psychic healing. This is where we hold our grief."

My heart. Love. Green. It was my mom's favorite color. She had a green car. I had tried to make it my favorite color, too, but it never really worked out. I thought of myself as more of a red girl, a fire girl. An image began to form in my mind, like a Polaroid developing. It was the interior of our old house. It was daytime, and no one was there. I had a POV as if I were a camera, standing in the corner of the dining room, looking into the foyer. I could see light streaming in over the sofa by the piano where no one ever sat. What was I looking at? With the green light shining on my heart, a feeling began to assemble there. It was so tremulous and powerful that I could feel my sturdily maintained stoicism start to crack. It wasn't depression exactly . . . more like, Eau de Sadness, with a few top notes of regret and confusion, a hint of helplessness . . . Ah, it was grief, in the form of a classical emotional wave. I told my brain to stop it, but my heart was controlling the tide. The emotion was roiling. I tried to suck it in, longing for a sturdy pair of head-to-toe emotional Spanx.

"What are you thinking about?" Barbara asked. I couldn't get the words together. I wouldn't have known what to say even if I could speak. "Let it out," she urged. I began to choke with sobs. They were unnamed, unspecific, but as they burst out they rocked me so hard that I couldn't breathe. She put a hand on my shoulder. "I think this is too much. I'm going to turn it off."

With a flip of the switch the light went off and the grief wave stopped. I breathed shallowly, regaining my composure. I could feel the cloth on my face soaked by my tears. A cool energy passed over me, as if someone had turned on a fan. Or a light switch. "This is the blue light on the fifth chakra, the throat charka," Barbara murmured. Ooh, it felt so calm and comfortable. "This is the seat of communication, how we express ourselves to others." No wonder I liked chakra number five so much; words worked for me! Talking. Writing. Expressing. Relief. I breathed for a few minutes, before Barbara covered my throat with the towel and pulled the wet washcloth from my face. Another flick. "Sixth chakra," she intoned. "Violet. The third eye. The vision you see." I didn't have any vision. I just felt calm. Barbara covered my eyes and flicked the switch one last time. "White light now, on your seventh chakra. The crown chakra. Your connection with the universe." What connection? There was no T-Mobile friends-and-family plan in my brain at the moment. My connection was wiped out. I was drained. I felt Barbara squeeze my hand. "Oh, Wendy," she sighed. "There are angels in this room."

The light show was over. I rested on the table. Barbara left the treatment room while I put my clothes back on. When I stepped out into the hall she was waiting for me and put her arms around me. "Let it out," she said. "You did a great job."

I stumbled back to Tracy and the Lotus House. I could lay the Psych 101 on my situation, but on some level what I experienced had no explanation. I knew the emotion was connected to the sadness I felt over the loss of my mother, a feeling that I certainly didn't like to acknowledge. If emotion was connected to detoxing, then it had to be connected to my health somehow. I didn't like that, either. Something happened on that table that went beyond explanation. I was a cynic, and yet I'd felt it. It led me to believe that there had to be a higher power, a deeper connection, something much, much bigger than Phil that would take a long time for me to understand. Tracy and I looped our arms together and walked back to the clinic one more time, for our final consultations with Dr. Rai.

Rai's office was decorated with red streamers, images of Hindu gods, and little golden elephants (representing, among other things, strength and longevity) all over the room. If nothing else, Ayurveda followers were festive. He had a few framed photos of his wife and children on the desk, as well as an eight-by-ten color photo of a tree. The tree was lit as though it had been photographed for the senior yearbook. Rai saw me checking it out. "That is my best friend," he explained.

I was so nervous. Still raw from chromatherapy, I again felt the trepidation that somehow Rai was the one who knew everything, and that I only had a few minutes to pry the future (the low-quantity, high-quality future) out of him. I wanted so much for him to hug me and say I was his favorite patient of the week, but he was very professional. He read over my chart, explained what I would need to do to follow up (brew this tea, eat that root, drink out of a silver cup, wear a silver ring on my left pinky finger that had a pearl in it that touched my skin). He also told me that there might be a problem with my ovaries, and I should have them checked out. Maybe that was the kid issue that had showed up astrologically? I wanted to clarify that whole "good life/long life" situation, and I asked him to look at my Jyotish chart. I had marked the grid with the explanations I'd found in one of the books in the Lotus House library, as if I could crack the ancient codes of foretelling and history with one night and an encyclopedia. Rai took a pencil and resketched my chart on a fresh piece of paper, filling in all those boxes with little dots. He pointed and nodded and finally looked up at me and sighed. This was it, the final note of my PK. "You must learn to forgive, Shan-kar," he offered up in a tender voice. "Until you forgive, you cannot heal."

The PK program ended on Friday afternoon. We planned to stay at Lotus Friday night. Tracy and I had booked one more night at a local hotel called Casas de Suenos before we flew home on Sunday morning. Ryan was on the same timetable so he decided to join us. When we got to the hotel, they only had a unit with a Jacuzzi, a couch, and one big bed, which meant that the three of us would have to share somehow. I couldn't juggle any *Three's Company* dynamics at the moment. Instead I sat down with my PK notes.

The biggest change—besides my attitude, apparently—was a shift in my eating. There were plenty of no's on the *pitta* balancing diet, including some likely suspects (bread, white sugar, alcohol, caffeine) and previously harmless culprits (bananas, brown rice, dairy, tuna, and oranges). On the yes list were lots of vegetables, couscous, beans, and berries. I didn't like the word *diet*. Diets had always gone very badly for me.

I was still trying to sort out a plan rationally, even though a little murmur deep inside reminded me that the insight on the chromatherapy table had nothing to do with rationality. I scribbled down a list of all the options I had picked up during the week, and whether I was going to take them:

## OPTIONS

| | |
|---|---|
| Take current Western meds | YES |
| Go to the gym | YES |
| Do yoga | YES |
| Eat modified Ayur diet | YES |
| Ayur food combo avoidance | ? |
| Follow *kapha* balancing diet | ? |
| No dairy from cows | YES |
| Drink rice milk | YES |
| Buy organic foods | YES (some) |
| Go back to regular dieting | NO |
| Take herbs | SOME |
| Take *triphala* (Ayur laxative) | YES |
| Take reg. laxatives | NO |
| Drink Ayur fiber | YES |

| | |
|---|---|
| Eat ginger/rock salt combo | YUCK |
| Drink hot water | YES |
| No more ice cubes | YES |
| "Evacuation" in a.m. | WILL TRY |
| Take Deep Love drops | YES |
| Drink Ayur wine | YES * |
| Do *nasya* (nose) drops | YES |
| Flush sinuses with neti pot | YES |
| Put cotton ball in ear | MAYBE |
| Early sleep/wake-up | NO WAY (9 p.m.—5 a.m.) |
| Modified sleep/wake-up | YES (12:30 a.m.—8 a.m.?) |
| Repeat wake-up prayer | YES |
| Clean face in a.m. | EASY |
| Scrape tongue | YES |
| Gargle with salt | NO |
| Chew seeds | NO |
| Use massage oils | NO |
| Burn incense | OK |
| Balance chakras | YES |
| Meditate | TRY |
| Study Ayurveda | YES |
| Go to therapy | YES |
| Acupuncture | TRY |
| Get body work | MAYBE |
| Explore Judaism | YES |

---

* Turns out it's not as good as red wine.

| | |
|---|---|
| Look into feng shui | YES |
| Cut off late-night phone calls with friends in L.A. | YES |
| Be quiet/still | YES (by 11 p.m.) |
| Take off nights for "me" | YES |
| Check ovaries | EVENTUALLY |
| Keep med chart | YES |
| Follow Andrew Weil | YES |
| Make goal list | YES |
| Ask for healing power | NOT YET |

I felt like my yeses included just enough to be challenging without going over. I had committed to way too many extreme diets and disappointed myself later when I couldn't stick with them. This time, especially when it came to food, I wanted to set reasonable expectations. The entire week of PK and travel cost about $3,500. I'd cashed out at the center's store with bottles of oils and sacks of herbs and some books about Indian gods and goddesses to keep me entertained on the plane. My suitcase smelled like sandalwood. *Everything* smelled like sandalwood.

That afternoon, the three of us shopped around Albuquerque's Old Town district. I'd never seen so many turquoise belt buckles in one place. It looked like George W. Bush's accessory drawer over there. We checked out an IMAX movie called *Creatures of the Sea*. We tried to have dinner in a normal restaurant but there was nothing we could eat. Not a lot of dal and ghee on the menu in your average joint. The following morning Ryan had the earliest flight; then Tracy had to fly back to San Fran. At her gate we hugged tightly, bonded in a special way by our experience. I had a couple of hours to kill before my flight took off for JFK. I wandered around the small airport. It was quiet on a Sunday morning, but there was still a cluster of hefty Americans eating cheeseburgers at the Burger King stand. There was nothing on my *pitta* (light, crunchy, spicy) diet to eat at the airport. I turned on my cell phone for the first time in a week and called my parents to let them know I was okay. I drank a liter of water at room temp, now that I understood cold water was off limits because it slowed down digestion. Then I stopped by the ladies' room to empty out before the flight.

When I sat in the stall I felt complete exhaustion roll over me. The intensity of the week and the drama of the last twenty-four hours overwhelmed me. "Forgive," Rai said. Who was I supposed to forgive? My mother, for dying? It wasn't her fault. Forgive myself? I hadn't done anything wrong. There was no one in particular looking for forgiveness from me. Besides, the research was inconclusive, but I was pretty sure I didn't get Wegener's granulomatosis from bearing a grudge. This was always the healers' contradiction: Disease isn't disease; it's dis-ease. It's not your body; it's you. But if forgiveness is what it takes to get better, why aren't hospitals packed with people apologizing, then walking out with clean bills of health? It wasn't an East versus West thing. I was armed with the science of allopathic medicine. I had opened my heart to options complementary medicine could provide. But I still didn't have a solid conclusion about the direction my treatment should take. Rai couldn't solve all my problems any more than Turner could. I'd have to keep looking for a cure.

I felt a cramp in my gut, a sensation I hadn't felt for weeks, then the tiniest release. In the bowl was a pellet about the size of a pea. It was barely anything, but it was something, and it could have been a gold nugget for the pride I felt in releasing it. It wasn't much when it came to "letting go," but it was a start.

# 7

# Beautiful Stranger

AUGUST 2001

Over that summer I attempted to continue the detox. A heat wave slammed New York City; my *pitta* constitution was so fried I had to detox from the detox. The meal planning was time-consuming and complicated, and I was back to sleeping no hours a night. My work at Oxygen continued to bounce back and forth between immense pleasure and ridiculous pressure. Oxygen had turned into my abusive boyfriend, slapping me in the face and then kissing and begging to make up and start over again. By the end of the summer I evaluated my life once again: I was almost thirty, fat, sad, and lonely, and still fighting Wegener's. I was barely pursuing alternative treatments; I had relapsed to what I called my "Candy and Precor Diet." It's very easy. You work out, go home, and eat candy. (If you're thinking it was high time for me to have a revolution in my body image thinking, you're right. It was soon to come.)

I looked for direction from the people I cared about, the passions I had, the things that made me happy . . . like my red nail polish and lipstick. Booze/Opium perfume/cigarette smell after a night on the town. My filing cabinets. Hot pink. Madonna and the *Buffy* musical. Glitter. Crystal bracelets. Chinese tins, TV shows, feminist pop culture books, brand-new magazines, design books, chocolate, labels and organization, Indian art, rubies and garnets, the set of keys I found in my mother's perfume bottle collection, black pinstripe pants, Peter Gabriel's voice, *Broadcast News*, *Tootsie*, *Amélie* and *Miller's Crossing*, the Upper East Side in movies, the Oriental cushions on my kitchen chair . . . and words.

Turns out it's really difficult to live an Ayurvedic life in the big city. I went back to do PK at the center two more times, once with Tracy and Sam (the three of us had a major detox together!), and once on my own. Each time it was less daunting and completely refreshing for my system. Each time I expected to score a perfect *vikruti* and get a pat on the head from Rai, but I never did. The closest he got was acknowledging, "You have suffered so much. Your real body is much different than the one you're in."

My second shot at chromatherapy was so emotional that the technician had to stop at chakra number three (I was a nervous wreck about it before I even walked in the room); the third time was so uneventful that I fell asleep. At Rai's suggestion, I eventually had my ovaries checked out; it turns out there was a minor hormonal issue that was an easy fix. I still use Ayurvedic lotions and oils. I am still a big believer in *triphala* and have done a home *basti* once or twice. Fine, twice. The *pitta* pacifying diet may be too intricate for me, but I try to follow the guidelines of avoiding foods (white sugar, white flour, processed foods, etc.) and food combinations (beans with cheese, eggs with milk, fruit with anything) that lead to systemic inflammation. I had the pearl ring made for me at an Indian jewelry store in Jackson Heights, Queens, because jewelry is always nice. I feel a lot more comfortable with yoga and chant the mantra that Rai designated for me (the Gayatri, meant to bring higher consciousness to the chanter, with a healthy dose of wisdom and understanding). At the bare minimum, I start every day with a prayer written by Ayurvedic doctor Vasant Lad:

> *Dear God, you are inside of me*
> *Within each bird, each mighty mountain*
> *Your sweet touch reaches everything*
> *And I am well protected.*
> *Thank you God for this beautiful day before me*
> *May joy, love, peace and compassion be a part of my life*
> *Today and every day.*
> *I am healing, and I am healed.* *

None of my private *mishegoss* seemed to matter after September 11, 2001. Our country, our world became a different place— sad and defiant—and New York City struggled to hold her head up proudly among the ruins. My responsibilities at the network

---

\* Vasant Lad, "The Daily Routine."

shifted from selfish to altruistic, then petered out. Right when I turned thirty, Oxygen gave me the boot. Defeated, exhausted, and determined to change my life, I finally booked a trip to the Duke Diet & Fitness Center, where I got over my fixation on weight loss. I was finally feeling good about what came naturally to my body. Eating well, exercising, and limiting stress was good strategy for every aspect of my health, including Wegener's. My body reset at a manageable weight, around 221 pounds. I was comfortable in my skin, proud of my body, and confident enough to write a book about it, called *The Fat Girl's Guide to Life*, scheduled for publication in April 2004.

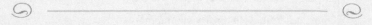

## NOVEMBER 2003

The Wegener's stayed normal and life went back to semi-normal. While I put the finishing touches on my book at night, I picked up a job at MTV writing for *Total Request Live*, or *TRL*, a live, daily video countdown show that catered to the screamiest audience possible: fans of Britney, Justin, and Beyoncé. I wouldn't be on staff, but "permalance." Since my COBRA benefits from Oxygen had run out, I'd continue to pay for my private health insurance at around $1,300 a month. It was my biggest expense, but I shuddered to think what would happen to me without insurance coverage (as so many Americans do). My new desk at MTV was just a few feet away from the cubicle where I'd started working in 1993. Almost everyone I worked with was younger than me. My favorite staffers included Joel and Elliott, the two writers who reminded me so much of the comedy boys I'd worked with during my first stint at MTV. After years laboring at women's magazines and women's television networks, it was a pleasure to be in a testosterone-fueled, take-it-or-leave-it male working environment, where men's mouths dropped open when Pamela Anderson sauntered into the studio.

I worked all day, tussled with the producers, then went out and partied with them at night. It was that sort of hell/fun that I could endure in my early twenties but was starting to give me a little wear and tear at thirty-two. So what if I was a little stiff in the morning, waking up after only a few hours of sleep. Big deal. That's what Aleve was for. So what if I couldn't always hear what people were saying to me. We worked with live bands and screaming fans. So what if the office cleaning lady caught me and Marta (reunited!) drinking a bottle of red wine we'd stashed in the filing cabinet . . . more than once. Those were long workdays! Besides, I didn't want my colleagues to know I was sick. When I started getting viselike headaches, I popped a Vicodin. More headaches, more Vicodin. I pictured myself as some sort of pain superwoman, withstanding more agony than the average girl could possibly take. It didn't strike me as unusual that by the middle of November I was taking ten to twelve Vicodin a day. I was still functioning perfectly well.

Then, on a November day before Thanksgiving, Madonna came to the studio. The execs asked me to produce her segments, knowing that I was a "fan" and had worked with her previously on awards shows. Tough call. I had gotten so bad at producing;

the adrenaline that used to turbopower me into thrillville now created unbearable stress that led to pain that led to . . . But it was Madonna. Like I was gonna say no?

She showed up tiny and nervous, surrounded by her team. Liz, her publicist, recognized me from the old days. I was worried since I looked so different now; though I had some post-Duke détente with my body, I was permanently puffed from the steroids. Liz was quite pleased that I'd made sure to provide Kabbalah water and champagne in the dressing room; Madonna had become an ardent follower of Jewish mysticism in the past couple of years, yet still desired a drop of liquid courage before her appearance. MTV honchos traipsed in and out of the studio, paying homage to the woman who had essentially made their careers possible. On the other side of the studio, I could barely see past the clouds of marijuana smoke pumping out of the dressing room of 50 Cent, a guest the same day. (I couldn't smell it, as the Wegener's was eroding my olfactory nerves, and my sense of smell had begun to fade.) He brought so many giant, tattooed, muscled, diamond-encrusted black men to the shoot that I wasn't sure which one was Fitty. Even though I was drenched in sweat, wearing a huge headset to communicate with the control room, I was relieved to discover I was still attractive enough to get hit on by enormous hip-hop entourage members. Hooray!

The ulterior motive of the MTV staff was to nudge Madge and Fitty together for a photo op, which somehow Ells and I managed. Madonna was trembling with nerves by the time she came on to premiere her video "Die Another Day" from her album *American Life.* Guess the champagne didn't take. It surprised me to think that anything unnerved Madonna, but I found it kind of endearing to know that a worldwide conqueror still got stage fright from time to time. Her repartee on the show was fabulous, as I expected. During the commercial break, she leaned over to me. I thought she might give me another much-needed pearl, à la "Be brilliant." But instead she whispered, "Is it okay if I say I want to give a shout-out to Eminem? We're from the same hometown." Me too, Madonna! I'm from Detroit, too! Never never never, while choreographing a dance routine to "Cherish" in my parents' basement in 1989, had I ever imagined Madonna asking my permission to say hi to Eminem on MTV. I assured her, "Go for it."

We made it through the crazy show, the celebs left the studio, and that night I collapsed in Marta's edit suite, crying and physically trashed. She ordered me to go home and rest. I climbed into bed fully clothed, without taking off my makeup. I was upset about looking and feeling shitty, and kind of despondent that Madonna didn't have a special message to share with me this time. Maybe she wasn't my guru after all.

Silly me, I didn't read into the message of the video she had chosen to premiere on the show that day: *I guess I'll die another day. It's not my time to go.*


The next two weeks weren't my finest. Since that exhausting Madonna day at the studio, my health/well-being/spirits, already fragile, sped steadily downhill. It wasn't fun to be me or be around me. I was torn between total meltdown and maintaining a stiff upper lip. It didn't help to be juiced back up to forty milligrams of prednisone per day, prescribed by Turner to combat some ongoing Wegener's symptoms. I couldn't sleep. I felt swollen, ugly, rotten. My hearing was getting worse, my nose was caving in, and my face ached with pain—clearly a total Wegener's flare.

I visited Allen, who decided to open up my eardrum by shooting a laser into it. Was this an Austin Powers movie or my life? If you think this sounds crazy, it absolutely is. He could numb the outer part of my ear, but not the eardrum itself. Well, a laser in your eardrum is as bad as you can imagine it would be. It seared a hole in my head. The beam didn't last long, but at least I had a standard by which to identify a 10 on the pain scale. I considered the possibility of a future full of lancing lasers and hearing aids. I couldn't believe this was my lot. At work, I moped past Mandy Moore and Angelina Jolie, filled with a lot of "Why me?" and some "Why this?" accompanied by the complete and utter ache of "Where is he???"—the guy who was supposed to be taking care of me. Why wasn't he here? What had I done to prevent him from showing up? Was Rai right—would I really not live a long life? I wondered when my attitude would change and some rah-rah would kick in. My whole book and my whole life would be screwed up if I were sick, deaf, and ugly. *C'mon, BTP, do I deserve this?*

By Thanksgiving weekend I could not function—my head felt like a giant was digging through it and squeezing my brain until it splooged between his fingers. I hadn't wanted to disturb my docs over a holiday weekend, but at 8 a.m. on Sunday I caved and called Allen. He sent me to the emergency room at Roosevelt. Deb sped out from Long Island to meet me there. I'd already started to decide who was going to get my stuff (Myrn could divvy up jewelry; Sam got Pee and Poo). I was almost certain that the pain in my head was a brain tumor. I begged a resident to take me out in a yard with a rifle and shoot me. He suggested I get some X-rays and CT scans instead. Smart proposition; there was inflammation in my head, and a nodule showed up in one of my lungs in the X-ray. As Arnold Schwarzenegger might say, "It's not a toom-ah." The diagnosis: a Wegener's flare and mastoiditis, an infection in the tiny bones behind the ear, had been causing the headache pain. The hospital gave me intravenous antibiotics, painkillers, and—a shocker—more steroids. They boosted me up to sixty milligrams of prednisone a day. I hadn't been prednisone-free for almost four years. Myrn flew in from Detroit on Sunday night. I didn't get out of the hospital until Tuesday afternoon, as I had to get an MRI scan of my brain to check for meningitis. I went directly to work at MTV. I was still taking eight Vicodin a day, and my headache still wouldn't quit.

DECEMBER 6, 2003

MY 32ND BIRTHDAY

**CURRENT BESTSELLERS:**
The Da Vinci Code *(fiction)*, The South Beach Diet
*(nonfiction)*; *won't be reading either*

**CURRENT CELEBRITY SCANDAL:**
*Michael Jackson was arrested for allegedly molesting
a twelve-year-old boy who has cancer*

**CURRENT FAVORITE MOVIE:**
Lost in Translation. *I think "Bill Murray" is*
*"Harrison Ford"*

**CURRENT GUILTY PLEASURE:**
The O.C.! *Long live Summer and Seth Cohen (as long*
*as she's Jewish or willing to convert)*

**IN MADONNA NEWS:**
*She's launching a line of dolls, apparel, and home décor*
*featuring the characters from her Kabbalah-inspired*
*children's book,* The English Roses

On the eve of my thirty-second birthday, I was at work in the MTV studio. The boys and I were planning to go out for drinks to celebrate later that night (no singing allowed). That's when the call came from Turner. "Are you sitting down?" he asked.

I slipped out of the control room and hunched down on a bench in the lobby. I jotted down notes on the back of a script for a Ludacris interview segment. "Go ahead."

"Okay. The Wegener's has flared, which is what led to your current state of exhaustion, hearing loss, and pain. It seems like the disease is destroying the cartilage in your nose, which as you've noticed, has become smaller and more upturned. We also found granulomas in your lungs and the outer layer of your brain, which is called the meninges. We're going to have to switch you to a much more aggressive chemotherapy, a drug called Cytoxan, to fight back. . . ."

I quietly left the studio without telling the boys I wouldn't be making it to my birthday party. I ignored their calls as they lit up on my caller ID. As I walked down the street, snow began to fall. I stopped at the drugstore on the way home to pick up the prescription Turner had called in, a pill that I would take every day. Cytoxan. Gwyneth had just found out that she was pregnant; I found out that the Wegener's had spread to both of my lungs and I had to get on Cytoxan ASAP. It was hardly the gift I wanted for my thirty-second birthday.

Turner felt confident that the drugs would be easily tolerated and send me swiftly into remission, but they made me so sick that I had to leave *TRL*. My superiors were unbelievably compassionate. By the time I came to the staff Christmas party I had gone through a major Cytoxan-induced makeover: I lost much of my hair, wore glasses to hide the slope in my nose, and walked slowly down the hall. Some of the staff members looked at me like I was a Make-A-Wish kid; their faces showed sympathy, but also a look of "That chick is done for!"

I didn't know what I was going to do about work, my book publicity, my friends, or maintaining my lifestyle. I didn't know what I wanted; I just knew that I was beyond bummed about it. A 50 percent chance of fertility loss from Cytoxan? Plus secondary cancer risks? Hadn't I made it clear way back when I was diagnosed that I was never going to be this . . . sick person, like Michele of the magnetic nose? Maybe I'd get cute again by the time I was thirty-five or thirty-six (if I made it that far), but shit—if I had a hard time getting a date now . . . wow. I didn't know what I had done to deserve this. I was tired of taking care of myself. I couldn't handle being strong for my parents, who had been so distraught when I told them about the latest turn in my treatment. I wasn't sure how I became this bitter, sick drama queen, toxic inside and out. What I wanted was simple: to be pretty, happy, and loved. Same as pre-Wegener's. I wished a therapist could simply fix me; I didn't have the energy to figure things out on my own. Somewhere deep inside I knew the key was to selflessly give, but oh God, I didn't have it in me now. I had to take care of myself, physically, mentally, especially now, and then address my deficiencies. I needed to tap into sweetness, graciousness, and compassion to bring it back to me. I couldn't believe I had to go through this. I'd had enough. Really. Enough.

Every morning at about 5:45 a.m. I'd hear the day's *Times* and *Post* slap up against my apartment door. That was my cue to pop my morning pills. It wasn't hard to wake up that early, considering I never went to sleep. I was amped out of my mind on prednisone. Up all night. Hallucinating. I spent a lot of time tracking the cycle of the sun and the moon. I would rouse before sunrise and put two thick white tablets out on the kitchen counter. I got down on eye level and examined them like diamonds. The four C's: Cytoxan, Cytoxan, Cytoxan, and Cytoxan. Every morning I actively chose to take those pills and make myself sick, in order to make myself well. I was relieved I didn't have to go to the hospital for infusions. The thinking was that I could either take a little chemo orally and be a little sick daily, or get infusions and be supersick once a week. Since most Wegener's patients respond well to Cytoxan (also known as cyclophosphamide), we went with option number one.

I received a profound gift in the mail from Carrie, who was living in Los Angeles. She had bedazzled a jewelry box and labeled each section with a day of the week, "AM/PM." It turned my pill popping from a painful situation to a reminder of love each time I cracked open the box. At least a dozen pills a day, including prophylactics (not condoms, but protective medicine; still I giggle every time I hear the word) that were supposed to protect me from the side effects of Cytoxan and the deficiencies it would cause in my immune system.

Within a day or two of starting the medication, I felt completely exhausted and my brain fogged up. The massive doses of steroids and surge of cortisol gave me moon face (just what it sounds like), bloated my already distended body, dusted a teenage nightmare of cysts all over my face and neck, and added a hump to my back. Prednisone retains fat and water where your body doesn't naturally have much of it: the sides of your face, tops of your feet, back of your neck, etc. The irony, of course, was that I was taking steroids as an anti-inflammatory. These complications were referred to as Cushing's syndrome, which was a fancy way of my body saying, "No more prednisone, please." "Cushing" sounded like "cushion" to me. I looked like a human pincushion. My 2Xs became 3Xs; my size 18s became size 22s. At my very Cushingest, my weight was 257. At 221, my body felt balanced. At 257, I felt like a beast.

The official list of side effects includes[*]:

Weight gain, particularly around your midsection and
    upper back
Fatigue
Muscle weakness
Rounding of your face (moon face)
Facial flushing
Fatty pad or hump between your shoulders (buffalo hump)
Pink or purple stretch marks (striae) on the skin of your
    abdomen, thighs, breasts, and arms
Thin and fragile skin that bruises easily
Slow healing of cuts, insect bites, and infections
Depression, anxiety, and irritability
Thicker or more visible body and facial hair (hirsutism)
Acne
Irregular or absent menstrual periods in females
Erectile dysfunction in males
High blood pressure

I never thought I'd be referred to in the same sentence as "moon face" and "buffalo hump."

I started drinking tremendous amounts of water to filter the drugs and ease my constant thirst. Worried about water purity (even though New York City tap water is the *best*!), I ordered

---

[*] http://www.mayoclinic.com.

cases of Poland Spring, drinking at least four liters a day at room temperature, per Dr. Rai's orders. When the drug cocktail really kicked in, each day ended up a pupu platter of low energy, nausea, unsettled sleep, funky appetite, bloating, and chemo brain. I had to do everything sooo slowly. Mick said over the phone, "This must be very hard on you, honey." I replied, "Yeah, but it could be worse," which was true. I could almost handle my physical degradation, since I knew it wouldn't last forever. But I was shocked every time I looked in the mirror: lethally unattractive. How was I going to promote a book in this situation?

Certainly the challenges I faced were nothing compared to my friend Amy's. We'd lost her back in October 2002, just before her thirtieth birthday. Now more than ever I had the deepest admiration for her feistiness, fighting the degradations of a hysterectomy, the pain of chemo ports, and the dubiousness of experimental halo radiation as her cancer spread. She had a black sense of humor and an honesty about the complete shitatiousness of her situation, remaining true to her acerbic nature until the very end. I looked to her example as a source of strength.

Each day I'd take my meds, make a little breakfast (usually oatmeal or something easy, because my digestion was getting screwed up), open the papers, and sit at the kitchen table while the sun came up. Then maybe I'd get back in bed for a while. It was dead winter. Icy, snow on the ground, and very little light. One post-Christmas morning I was sitting at the table with my Cinnamon & Spice reading "Page Six" when I suddenly felt lightheaded. I heard a sonic hum and the world turned black and white. I recalled this feeling—I was about to faint. The same thing had happened to me once when I was a teenager on a summer trip to Israel, partying in Tel Aviv, drinking no water but lots of cocktails, standing on a packed bus in the desert heat. The world went black and white, I passed out, and woke up with my head hanging out the bus window on Dizengoff Street. That's what I needed—air would make me feel better. I went to my kitchen to heave open the window a crack. That's all I remember. When I came to, I was lying faceup in the hallway between my bathroom and my bedroom. Wow, I thought, I've never seen my chandelier from this position. So pretty and sparkly up there! Hmm, what's that? A bloody handprint on the wall. And a smear of blood sliding down next to it . . . Wait. Is that *my* handprint? I put my hand to my face. When I pulled it away, it was covered with blood. Slowly I lurched up and looked in the bathroom mirror. I had a vertical gash about two inches long between my eyes. My forehead was already beginning to bruise and swell. I also had a pretty big bump on the back of my head. Shaking, I washed off my hands and shuffled back to the kitchen to see if I had anything in the freezer that resembled ice to ease the swelling. No peas; a box of Birds Eye frozen broccoli florets would have to do the job. The kitchen window was still open, but the radiator cover beneath it looked like it had been kicked in and scraped. Calling on my best Nancy Drew skills, I realized that I must have opened the window, fainted, and fallen forward, gashing my head on the corner of the window and the radiator cover. Then I'd gotten up and walked toward the bathroom, leaning against the wall (ergo, stamping it with a handprint like the one on "Wilson" the soccer ball in *Cast Away*) and slid down to the floor, smacking the back of my head and fainting faceup. My oatmeal was rock solid. The apartment was freezing. The sun was up. I'd been out for at least a few minutes. Wrapped in a hand towel to mop up the blood, I put the box of broccoli on my face and crawled back into bed. What to do now? I called my parents, who happened to be in New York that weekend to celebrate New Year's Eve in Times Square and check up on me. Myrn answered the phone.

"Hi, no big deal but I think I fainted and hit my head." I unlocked my apartment door while Myrn rushed over in a cab, then got back in my bed. She freaked when she entered the bedroom and saw me. "Oh, my God!" she shrieked, "It's like you have a vagina on your face!" She was right. The wound was pretty Cronenbergian.

Myrn called a friend who knew a lot of local plastic surgeons. What I really needed to do was go to an emergency room, but with my immune system crushed from the Cytoxan and the prednisone, a germy holiday ER would not be an ideal place to hang out. I called Turner's office. He was away on vacation. (See! Do *not* get sick at Christmas!) Luckily Dr. Baker, my original caretaker, was covering for him. He instructed me to get to his hospital's ER immediately. Mick came by and picked us up in a cab. Dazed, we crossed an iced-over Central Park to go to Mount Sinai Hospital.

I was taken through triage fairly quickly, then parked on a stretcher in one of those little curtained cubicles. When another stretcher rolled up nearby, the corner of it nudged my curtain open. I saw a foot that looked like it belonged to one of the monsters from *Where the Wild Things Are*. Someone had better amputate that gangrenous thing—it looked like it was about to fall off. Hopefully not on my stretcher.

A young doc came by to examine my wound. "How many stitches will I need?" I asked as he bent over me.

"No stitches necessary. I'm just going to go ahead and adhere this together with some liquid bandage." Excuse me? Gaping wound on my face! You could practically see my skull! This called for more than a squirt of superglue. My parents, God bless 'em, told Baby Doc that we were going to wait for a plastic surgeon. We waited. No big, as it would take a while to be admitted to the hospital to be tested and find out if heart irregularities, vasovagal episodes, fluid in my ears, or mastoiditis had caused me to pass out. The plastic surgeon on call specialized in hand surgery. Not ideal, but it was certainly a step up from melted Band-Aids. He took out a tiny wooden box with his needles and sutures in it. I watched him stitch together my forehead in a mirror. He did an excellent job, but I'll always have the trace of a Harry Potter scar running down the center of my forehead. Dr. Rai would probably say that my third eye had been split right open. Now I'd probably never have a shot at higher consciousness, no matter how many times I chanted that Gayatri.

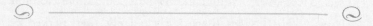

JANUARY 2004

Stitched up, unemployed, and quarantined from others' germs in my apartment, I started Dapsone, a prophylactic (hee, hee) drug meant to protect me from contracting pneumonia while my immune system was being compromised. My mouth and lips blew up; my tongue swelled with blisters. An allergic chemical burn seared the skin on my torso, arms, and legs. I looked like a cheeseless pizza. I would open all the windows to the winter cold and take all my clothes off—it hurt to even wear a robe—and still feel boiling hot. It itched like crazy and lasted for almost three weeks.

My doctors knew I was allergic to sulfur from that long-ago Bactrim episode; there was no way I had been prescribed a sulfa drug, right? Wrong. They forgot. Dapsone was indeed a sulfa drug. So why was it prescribed in the first place? For the classic reason: "protocol." Three antibiotics were added to prevent the burn from evolving into Stevens-Johnson syndrome, a disease that causes your skin to peel off. The drug I used to replace Dapsone made me so nauseous that I threw it up. No more prophylactics.

We added Valium and Restoril to keep me from weeping at least three times a day, moving through steroid-inspired cycles of mania and despair. Nutty and paranoid, I began to see little starfish people (like that little peachy one in *Finding Nemo*) dancing around my friends' faces on the rare occasions that anyone came by. Some people long for company when they're sick, but I felt shitty and antisocial, and the last thing I wanted was other people wallowing around in my cloud of misery. My book publisher called to see if I could do a photo shoot to accompany the excerpt that was going to run in *Self*. I didn't want them to know I was such a wreck, and might not be able to promote the book. "I can't," I said weakly, drumming up an excuse. "I'm . . . in Florida."

My hair fell out—but not evenly. It was more like I lost clumps from the top of my head. I balanced it out by growing more fuzz on my arms, shoulders, and face. I wasn't sick enough to die, but I wasn't well enough to live my normal life. I also feared that the treatment was worse than the disease. With all this chemo, I could be kissing my fertility good-bye while opening myself up to a lifetime of secondary cancers and other systemic disorders. My ob-gyn tossed Ortho Tri-Cyclen in the mix to regulate my hormones and try to cling to a monthly period, 'cause when you're already a walking drug cocktail . . . why not?

My usual exercise routine of gym time—something that kept me sane as well as fit, if not thin—went out the window (probably the one where I sliced open my face). It was all I could do to shuffle from my bed to my bathroom. Plus the Cytoxan killed my taste buds. Everything tasted like sandpaper. The only thing that I enjoyed imbibing—a massive pleasure that has never gone away—was bubbles. Carbonation became my drug of choice. In my whole life I never cared about soda . . . but now? Heaven was a can of Canada Dry diet ginger ale. Actually, any kind of ginger ale. And Izze sodas. Nothing better than a grapefruit Izze in a can. Paradise was the natural fruit soda section at Whole Foods. I tried to find sodas flavored with real sugar or juice to avoid artificial sweeteners (I'd also discovered I had a nasty Splenda allergy). I would add seltzer to anything. Seltzer in juice, in coffee, in tea. It was my only vice. Friends and family sent me baskets of food that I couldn't enjoy. The only tastes I could stand were cheese and ice cream. So I ate a lot of cheese and ice cream, because I could taste them and because I was miserable, and to deprive myself of cheese and ice cream at that point felt like insult added to serious injury. My weight ballooned. I went from a 38DDD bra to a 42G bra—G as in "Oh, my God, my Gazoons are Gargantuan." I left my apartment for an hour each week to see a psychiatrist who specialized in patients with chronic illness, but my synapses were too shot to be able to process intellectual talk therapy. I convinced her to prescribe me some antidepressants instead.

I looked in the mirror at a bloated, scarred, fuzzy, balding, pug-nosed monster and no longer saw myself. All the encouragement and advice about positive body image that I'd written about in *The Fat Girl's Guide to Life* just months before felt like lies. I could find no beauty, no self-respect. Just when I had come to peace with my body, that treaty was broken by this evil, Nazi disease.

People often ask me how they ought to act when a friend reveals she's been diagnosed with a serious illness. Generally they respond to their pal in one of two ways: plug in, or freak out. Plugger-inners would rather err on the side of doing too much for a sick friend than too little. Freaker-outers worry about screwing up an unspoken code of behavior, or fear that somehow they'll contract a disease themselves. There is a third category of respondent, a kind of illness voyeur who seems to get a perverse thrill from your bad luck. It's like schadenfreude, but more like *sickenfreude*. These folks almost feel pleasure when you become weak or dependent. For the most part you wonder why you were friends with them in the first place. I say, Nuke 'em. End those relationships. No poisonous energy needed now, thank you very much.

I was shocked by how clueless some people became when speaking to me about illness and disease. It may have been their nerves talking, but I was mystified by acquaintances who compared another's scourge to my own. Ah, the foolish things even the most well-intentioned people say:

"I don't know what to say!" (How about, "I heard and I care"?)

"But you *sound* okay."

"Chemo drip? At least it wasn't a porto-cath."

"That's nothing. My sister-in-law's mother's brother got bitten by a scorpion, and. . . ."

"You have [INSERT ILLNESS HERE]? Well, I know how you feel because I broke my leg when I was seven."

"I know how you feel. My cat had leukemia."

"I know how you feel. I have symptoms of lupus. It's not *actual* lupus, but it's still pretty intense."

Basically any sentence that starts with "I know how you feel" is not a fantastic opener. Also unwelcome: visitors with colds. I know you want to show up for me, but don't you know better? I have a completely compromised immune system. That means it doesn't work. Your sneeze will become my pneumonia. Thanks for coughing on me. Now excuse me while I go Purell my entire body.

Then there's the whole contingency of silver lining-ers who can't make psychic room for the possibility of unwellness. They say things like:

"Well, look at the bright side . . ."

"Well, at least you still have all ten fingers."

"Well, at least it's not cancer."

At least it's not cancer? Cancer has funding for research.* Cancer has cures. People have heard of cancer. I'm almost jealous of cancer. Autoimmune disease may be different than cancer, but no one should have to suffer through either one.

Sometimes during a casual conversation, a friend will say something like "Oh, I had the worst flu . . ." then cut themselves off in embarrassment. "I can't believe I'm complaining about the flu after everything you've gone through!" Don't feel too guilty. I hear myself bitching about my sore joints or funky nose and then think, There are so many people worse off than me. Why am I kvetching? Everyone has a different scale of suffering. But if you're wondering . . . you're right. Compared to whatever's bugging you, mine is probably much, much worse.

Still, I say it's better to attempt to connect than avoid. If you're not sure what to say, I'll offer up a script, an illness Mad Lib of sorts. While all outreach is welcome, personally, I prefer a phone call. If you must write, send a truly thoughtful e-mail or a handwritten card. So old-fashioned, I know, but it's a valuable memento for your sick pal to hold on to while she wallows in bed watching repeats of *Montel*.

Okay, the script:

---

* "About 860 cancer drugs are being tested in clinical trials, according to the pharmaceutical industry's main trade group. That is more than twice the number of experimental drugs for heart disease and stroke combined, nearly twice as many as for AIDS and all other infectious diseases combined, and nearly twice as many as for Alzheimer's and all other neurological diseases combined." Andrew Pollack, "For Profit, Industry Seeks Cancer Drugs," *New York Times*, September 1, 2009.

*Please leave a message after the beep.* (This is the other thing—don't expect your friend to pick up the phone if she's feeling rotten. Caller ID to the rescue, once again.)

"Hi, [PATIENT'S NAME], it's [YOUR NAME]. I heard about your [SICKNESS SITUATION]. I'd really like to help you, but I'm not sure how. If you want to hang out, or if I can bring you food or something, I'd be really happy to. But for now, I just want to say that this sucks, and I'm thinking about you, and you don't have to call me back. The end."

The point is to tell your loved one that you're aware and you care (same goes for any bad news—job loss, breakup, death of a parent). Don't assume you'll have to hang out in hospital waiting rooms or change bedpans. Use your personal skill set to help your friend. If you love music, make your pal a great CD. If you have a car, offer a pickup or a drop-off at a doctor's office. If you have cash, by all means, buy an expensive gift. All efforts are appreciated. There are plenty of ways to show your love without impersonating Florence Nightingale.

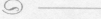 

FEBRUARY 2004

Research showed that only 15 percent of Wegener's patients on Cytoxan lost their hair. Even with my mediocre math skills, I could deduce that gave me an 85 percent chance to be coiffure safe. About a month into the treatment, sitting in my favorite perch—on my couch watching the new TV my parents had gifted me during my incarceration—I noticed a few fine hairs on the throw pillow. I started absentmindedly stroking my head and in a couple of days I'd collected a little hair nest on the floor. It was an EEG test that finally did my hair in. I needed to get my brain waves measured to make sure mine hadn't melted during the whole slip-'n'-slide, forehead slice and dice (we never did determine exactly what went wrong). The test involved attaching a couple of dozen pods to my scalp with some sticky goo. The pods looked like those wax earplugs that nerdy kids at the swimming pool used to wear; I had to wear them in my ears whenever I took a shower. The technician plugged the pods into a machine, turned it on, and got a readout. My brain was just fine. But when she pulled the pods off, clumps of hair came with them. It took me forever to get the leftover pod gunk out of my hair when I got home. It was the stereotypical shower scene from a movie, where the showerer starts out shampooing her hair very industriously and then ends up crying in the stall, sinking down the tiles, the water indistinguishable from her salty tears. Very *Silkwood*.

Before I went through it, hair loss always seemed like a small price to pay for a healthy body. I couldn't understand why cancer patients got so rattled by it. It's hair. It grows back. Aren't you glad you're surviving? Who cares what you look like? But when I lost it, it was like I lost myself. Another blow to my ego when I was pretty trashed already. Plus I didn't look bald and *cute*. I had half a head of hair—the lower half. I looked like Britney in the middle of her infamous head shave. I tried a Giuliani-type comb-over move to disguise my new male-pattern baldness. Some fellow chemo takers suggested I go completely bald, but I certainly wasn't going to shave what I had left, not when there was a strand or two worth saving. Reality check: I would never look like one of those fierce women who can pull off a sexy *Star Trek* alien dome, or an ambiguously gay rock star who can carry off a brush cut.

I finally got a little honesty from Dorothy, my genius hairstylist. I figured she could trim my classic bob haircut a bit to give me the tiniest sense of style until it all went and I'd have to wear a wig. Dorothy looked at me in horror when I shuffled into the salon. "What's *wrong* with you?" she demanded in her Polish accent, eyeballing my poofy face and bandages. I gave her the health update. She poked at my listless strands for a few minutes before she finally gave up. "I'd straight-iron, but why bother?" She shrugged. I laughed my ass off, so grateful for someone offering a truth without a Pollyanna-like cheer. When I got home, she and her assistant Manal sent me a lush bouquet of flowers.

I needed a new look, so I started simple, modeling myself on Rosie the Riveter with her badass red bandana. The head wrap looked majorly goofy to me, so I tried to amp it up with big hoop earrings—take it from homemaker to hip-hop. No good. With my face bloated and pasty from the meds, all I needed was a tiny blue tear tattooed under my eye to officially make me look like a member of an East L.A. girl gang: "'Eyyy, how you doin', Chemolita?" I threw a jaunty cap on top of the head scarves, hoping to pull a

Missy Elliott, but just looked like a grandpa. Definitely time to upgrade to a different head covering. I needed a wig.

I called my friend Gaby, a young breast cancer survivor. She informed me that wigs were pricy, but it was too important to skimp. I thought it would be easy to artificially re-create my silent movie star bob-with-bangs look, because everyone thought I was wearing a wig anyway. It was the same style that actresses wear when they play strippers in a movie—then they pull off the wig and their unnatural blond extensions cascade out. But a fourteen-dollar hot pink Ricky's bob wasn't going to cut it for me. Gaby sent me to a serious wig store on the Upper West Side called Barry Hendrickson's Bitz-N-Pieces (bald chicks—always suckers for funky spelling!). When you're buying the real deal, it's not a walk-in situation. I had to call and make a reservation ahead of time, as if I were going to a hair salon. Which I was. A hair salon without the heads attached.

I'd walked past Bitz-N-Pieces a million times without registering it. It was on the second floor of a building near Columbus Circle, a major Broadway intersection. Brightly lit and mirrored, it looked like a relic from another time (early 1960s?) and another place (Miami Beach?). Who was buying these flips and falls and fur hats? Um, I was.

Gaby's warning was an understatement. Wigs are *expensive*—they can cost thousands of dollars. Guess when you need one (cancer sufferer, Orthodox Jewess, Star Jones), you need one. So wig masters charge what the market will bear. Turner had given me a prescription for a wig, hoping my insurance would cover some of the expense. Good luck with that. They also rarely cover hearing aids.

I walked in at the designated time with a photo of myself and gamely announced, "I want a wig that looks like my old hair." I know there are women who declare, "As long as I'm doing this, I'm gonna go blond/short/curly/wispy!" à la Samantha in *Sex and the City*, but that wasn't me. I just wanted to look like myself. I hadn't spent my entire adult life rocking a hairstyle to give up on it just because of stupid Wegener's granulomatosis. The salesman (who, sadly, was not Barry Hendrickson himself) brought out wigs in different shades and lengths and then put me in an alcove that looked a lot like a Broadway star's dressing room. Big mirror, bright bulbs, and a countertop with a big brush and a hand mirror on it.

My biggest challenge was trying not to wig out. (Come on, I can't resist.) My *pitta*-powered fury rumbled. I wanted to lash out at every employee in my eye line. I'm sure I wouldn't have been the first customer to do it, either. No one wants to be in a situation where some poor Indonesian lady's hair is your must-have, but it wasn't their fault I had to come a-shoppin'. I was sure the staff was familiar with tonsorial rage. That was probably why they left me alone in the dressing room while I tried on my new fake dos.

When I selected a shoulder-length wig that most looked like my hair color, a guy named Furio came in to cut and style it for me. I didn't know they were going to do that. I was like a real-life Barbie head. He kept trimming off little . . . well, little bitz and pieces and asking for my opinion. I thought those bitz were too little. Every go-round made me more angry and resentful. I finally snapped, "Can't you just hack away at the thing?"

Insulted, he leaned over and whispered urgently in my ear, "I'm just trying to build *trust.*"

I walked out of the store into the omnipresent winter deep freeze with my six-hundred-dollar (!!!) wig on my head, the cheapest one they had. I was sure that everyone would point and stare at me. No one did. I looked like a somewhat religious Jewish woman, not an uncommon sight on the Upper West Side of Manhattan. Figuring I should live it up during this rare time out of my apartment, I swallowed my germ nerves and went to a nail salon across the street. I hadn't had a manicure since my birthday, when the whole Cytoxan drama began. When I reached for my color, Bordeaux (Essie No. 12), my hand faltered. I couldn't do it. I couldn't wear my signature nails or my signature lipstick when I didn't have my signature hair, signature face, or signature body. Maybe nails were just nails to a regular girl, but to me, my manicure was an essential part of my identity. I remembered going to the nail salon with my mother when I was a little girl. She went every week to have her nails done, and they always looked fabulous. Trembling, I moved away from my traditional red and chose Raspberry No. 89 instead. It was a monumental moment, when I officially stashed my "self" away, hidden inside a body that didn't make sense to me anymore.

# 8

# What It Feels Like for a Girl

As I tried to fight back from the disease and the treatment, three things became very obvious:

- Everyone knew someone with something similar to what I had.
- Everyone knew the way to fix what I had.
- Everyone was going to tell me exactly how to do it.

This left me feeling incredibly defensive, that same kind of vulnerable vibe I get when a yenta type asks, "So . . . are you seeing anyone?" She's just chomping at the bit for me to say, "Not really." Instantly she knows the perfect guy for me and is determined to set us up. Hell, he might not even be the perfect guy . . . but damn it if he's not good enough! "What the hell are you waiting for, Wendy—perfection? This is your *life partner*. You can't be so choosy, or those ovaries of yours are going to start kweefing dust. With all these drugs . . . who knows what's happening down in your lady areas? Chop-chop, girl!"

Sick love is a problem. I don't mean being so in love that you're sick over it; I'm talking about being sick and finding love. Deathly illness is the perfect time to already have a husband— Brad, or Kyle, or TJ or whoever, doing his best to get you through the night. What a relief to know someone has already signed a document saying he's going to stick with you no matter what (well, around 50 percent of the time, based on current statistics). When you're sick, you become needy in a way that trumps anxiety or fear of a lifetime of loneliness. It's not only that you want a TCB (taking care of business, every day) type of guy, or that you need a partner in crime to help you feed the kids and pay the bills. Many women with chronic or fatal illnesses have told me that what they want most from their partner is simple: "Make the bed." Hear that, fellas? *Make the frickin' bed.* Sometimes that's literally what we need, but it's also the idea of him taking care of the little things (without being told) so you don't have to. Above and beyond that, you hope for a partner who is legally bound to tell you how beautiful and wonderful you are while you're yakking mystery meds into the toilet. Someone to hold you during those endless dark nights when you're wired on steroids, sleeplessly convinced that tiny fairies are living in your lingerie drawer. You need a husband's name and number to fill in as your emergency contact. 'Cause if it ain't him, then it might end up being your parents, and the last thing you want to do is call Mom and Dad when you're twenty/thirty/forty years old and freaking out. So if you're like me, still on the hunt when the Big Bad arrives? Uh-oh.

Of all the times that I didn't feel sexy and couldn't get my flirt on, the Cytoxan Cycle topped the list. The meds killed my sex drive. I kept waiting for that Lifetime movie moment when I would be about to board a bus, wearing a head scarf and weeping, and some hot guy (for casting purposes, let's say Kelly Ripa's husband, or for Wendy purposes, I'm good with Jon Hamm from *Mad Men*) would run in, gently peel the Pucci scarf off my head, kiss me passionately, then cut to the "Whoa, those were tough times!" wedding toasts a year later as the band played Kool & The Gang's "Celebration." That moment did not arrive.

I felt ugly and raw. I'd stay up all night watching Discovery Channel specials about six-hundred-pound moms and the lady who was just a torso but somehow managed to get married and have two kids anyway. A very efficient way to make myself feel even more loserish. Someone wanted to procreate with a torso but I couldn't even get kissed? There was a guy swooning in front of a six-hundred-pound vagina, but nobody loved me?

I had lots of men in my life, but they all wore white coats and made me call them "Doctor." While other women my age were wearing sexy sheaths and collecting digits, I was wearing a paper gown and giving urine samples. This was not what my female family members were talking about when they advised me to "land a doctor," though the process of finding the right physician is a lot like dating. M.D. Date. Finding Dr. Right. (Note: Dr. Right can most certainly be a woman, but just roll with the analogy here.) The dream shifts a bit: you no longer have to marry the guy; you just have to find one who is accepting new patients. Meeting the perfect doc—the one who understands you, who has a personality you like, who listens, who takes out the garbage . . . No, no, Wendy, a mate takes out the garbage. See, I get confused! But follow my logic: You start out knowing you need a special person in your life. You ask around, see if anyone knows someone who might be compatible. Friends make recommendations. You find a window in your schedule and then meet for the first time. You select an outfit that you hope he will find appealing. You hope he'll find you special—somehow more compelling than the others. You go over your notes—the stories you'd like to tell, the questions you want to ask, your painful doctor/patient relationship history up to this point. Sometimes you know it's a disaster from the start; "Have you always had that bald spot?" is a rough way to start a conversation, especially if you didn't think you had one. Sometimes you feel him but he blows you off ("Let's see, I have to go to the Congo with Doctors Without Borders to repair a few cleft palates, but I have an appointment available . . . seventeen and a half months from now"). But sometimes it's just right. There's compatibility, even a chemistry, which makes you trust the person sitting across from you the first time you meet him, believing that he'll get you through the biggest challenge of your life.

Then you pay him, but that's a different story.

When I look back on all the time, effort, and drama that went into managing my health situation, I'm vexed that that particular time, effort, and drama did not go into managing a husband situation. I shared the dating dilemmas of my peers; it's just that many of mine took place while I was under sedation. Sometimes I still look up when a doctor enters the room and I think, Are you my otolaryngologist, or is that just a laryngoscope in your pocket?

FEBRUARY 2004

Desperate to pretend nothing unusual was going on while undergoing chemotherapy, I took a freelance writing gig with a new client. The job was a disaster. I was too tired and spaced-out to do the work, and had no energy left over to negotiate new personalities and conflicts. Again, I remind you, massive steroids and managing moods do not mix. I told myself to stay calm, not to worry about what people would think of me if I wasn't working or going out to dinner. Dial it down. Stop feeling guilty and worried about repaying everyone for their generosity and equaling things out. No one knew what I was doing in my apartment every day (watching crappy cable) and no one cared (in a nice way). I had to keep it simple and remind myself that it was okay to blow off anything, especially at that time.

Watching the tube, nothing irritated me more than the episode of *Sex and the City* when Samantha chucked off her cancer-induced wig in a moment of triumph. I don't think so. Bald is only beautiful for Seal and that model with the crazy tattoo on her scalp. Also, Carrie (the character whom I was supposed to relate to the most according to the quiz on HBO's website, though I felt more like a Miranda) constantly intimated to the at-home audience that if you're not with a man, you might as well be dead. Hello, Carrie? Mr. Big is death. Mark my words, he's the kind of guy who will dump you on your wedding day. Huh. Maybe my heath issues were providing me with a shortcut, an express lane for savvy girls to scoot past shitty relationships.

With ten weeks of treatment down and two to go, I worried that my doctors would make me continue on Cytoxan if we didn't start to see some major improvement. The numbers still weren't fantastic. I wasn't feeling much better, though by this point I was beginning to understand that my gut instinct was an essential diagnostic tool. As if I weren't already the Mayor of Fugly Town, one of my eyes started bulging out of my face. An ophthalmologist who bore a distinct resemblance to a Filipino Doogie Howser told me it could be proptosis due to Wegener's. Oh, fantastic. Apparently I also had early signs of cataracts in both eyes, likely caused by the high doses of prednisone. I was uncomfortable and exhausted, tired of being a good sport. I wanted my life back. I had a message for my Wegener's. I wanted to announce, "Yo, Wegs, it stops here. Leave the eye sockets alone. No spreading to my throat, you understand? Keep my kidneys out of it. While we're at it . . . attention all powers that be: I refuse to let Wignahuh's Shamalattatadingdong take me down. Not going to happen. I already lost my nose, my hearing, my hair, and my sanity. My head is killing me. I've got gunk in my lungs and a serious case of googly eye. That's enough. We're done." But it was like one of those bad dreams when you're being attacked and screaming as loud as you can, and no sound comes out.

My brain finally checked out. I flipped the switch from

"Wow, this situation sucks" to "Hey, I'm never getting out of bed again."

When I first got sick, my friends assured me I was strong and brave for pursuing treatment and trying to maintain my usual lifestyle. I simply saw no other choice. Now I know that I could have simply gotten addicted to painkillers, or tried to throw myself off a roof. Instead I discovered a third option: deep and permanent bonding with my side-sleeper pillow, bra-free, twenty-two hours a day. I wanted to avoid undergarments, eat carbs, and ignore everyone. I spent five weeks in bed, just lying there and staring out the window. Even Madonna songs couldn't cheer me up. It was like having "Frozen" stuck on permanent replay. I didn't answer the phone, didn't reply to e-mails, and didn't leave my house. Every once in a while a friend or neighbor would drop off food, and you can pretty much have anything delivered in New York. Eventually I dragged myself to another shrink to get some kick-start antidepressants. Mostly I watched reruns of *Felicity*—I'd TiVo'd four seasons' worth and watched them in chronological order. I felt as bad as Felicity did when she was crushed by the love of her life, Ben. I was completely invested in Felicity's life (running for student council, working at Dean & DeLuca) because she was the only thing getting me through. Would she ultimately pick bad-boy Ben (Don't do it!) or good-guy Noel (Yes, yes!)? Would she listen to her heart and become an artist, or listen to her parents and go pre-med? Felicity and her friends were the only things keeping me connected to normalcy. Which wasn't very normal.

MARCH 2004

At the end of an extension to fifteen weeks, victory. Turner switched me from Cytoxan to Imuran, an immunosuppressive drug sometimes used to help prevent the body from rejecting organ transplants. Sam scooped me out of my apartment for a celebratory trip to South Beach, which was sunny and sweet but not much fun. My head was still killing me. I'd tapered down to seventeen milligrams of prednisone, but had to bump back up to forty milligrams a day, along with handfuls of Vicodin, Percocet, and Darvocet to manage the headache pain.

I kept busy with an episode of vertigo (kind of like being on a boat in stormy seas, except *not*), which was resolved after ten days with a drug called Antivert and a decision to get new tubes implanted in my ears. The tube implant had been way too painful to do in the ENT's office the last time we tried, so I'd have to go under general anesthesia in the hospital. The night before surgery I got my period. (Every time I got it, I did a little tribal dance of relief. Period here! I am woman! I'm still fertile! Maybe I'll give birth to a dragon, but at least the possibility exists!) In a rolling bed outside the operating room, all dolled up in hospital gown chic, I waited for what felt like forever. No magazines to page through, no e-mail to read. Just plenty of time to get nervous over nothing. I finally waved over a nurse. "What's the holdup?"

"We need you to take a pregnancy test."

"Actually . . . I have my period." *Actually . . . I haven't exactly felt like getting my sexy on while my body exploded and my hair fell out.*

"I know, but it's protocol," said the nurse, brushing me off.

"But I'm literally bleeding. I'm chock full of tampon!" I protested.

"Prrrr-otocol!" she trilled. An hour and a half after I peed in a cup and proved my womb empty, I finally went into surgery.

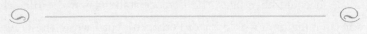

APRIL 2004

My premiere book reading would be the first time in months that I'd see many of my friends and colleagues, including the publishers of *The Fat Girl's Guide*. My nose had completely caved in and I needed to buy a pair of glasses to hide the deformity. A few days before the release, I stepped out to shop for an outfit to wear to the reading. I was chilling in a long line at Lane Bryant behind a lot of other fat ladies. Even in New York, sartorial options are limited when you're in the size 22 zone. I glanced at a mannequin wearing the cutest striped bra and panties. Pow! I fell in love with that mannequin, like something straight out of a Jon Cryer movie. She was just a torso, but she was thick and sexy and I thought, I wish I could take her home. She looks great. I scrutinized the women behind the counter and the women in line at the store, and thought, I want to take them home, too. Their bodies looked so appealing to me. They looked luscious. They looked healthy. They looked like me, minus months

of drug drama and a wig. Yes, they were sweaty, harried, and im-
patient, and some had crazy nails and Lil' Kim eyebrows, but
every one was beautiful in her own way. Fat *and* beautiful. Completely desirable. I mused, Who better to touch than me? What
better body to hold than mine? Why does a thin woman deserve
love any more than I do?

*Duh. She doesn't.*

In that moment, I understood why I wrote *The Fat Girl's
Guide*. It could have been the Percocet talking—at the time, I
was jamming on a whole lot of Percocet—but I wrote the book
because I wanted to connect with everybody, on a physical and
emotional level. It was a book about touching and being touched
without fear, which was especially potent for someone who hadn't
been able to touch anyone for almost four months. I couldn't
allow Wegener's to invalidate the progress I'd made when it came
to thinking about fat and body image in a positive way.

I wore my LBs (hmm, Lane Bryants = lbs. = pounds) and my
fake-out glasses to the reading at a Barnes & Noble in Greenwich
Village, followed by a packed reception thrown by my friend
Sue. Deb set up readings and events on Long Island. I tried to
swallow my insecurity about the way I looked and simply be in
the moment, surrounded by people who cared about me. Let them
think my sick fat was regular old *fat* fat. Luckily the book got
wonderful press, reviews, and feedback. I did a zillion radio interviews, then flew to Michigan for a blowout reading at a Borders
in West Bloomfield, where half the people I grew up with showed,
including my first-grade teacher from Pine Lake Elementary
School. I was so wiped that I slept in the car on the way to the

bookstore and back. Mick and Myrn threw a beautiful kosher dinner in my honor at our house, and even ordered a cake that looked like the cover of my book. I think chunks of it are still in their freezer. I was interviewed on CNN, and appeared on *The View* all bloated and wearing my wig. I threw up in a wastebasket in my dressing room on the way out of the studio.

As ever, I was endlessly grateful for the support I received. Mick and Myrn and Josh took excellent care of me, along with all my pals. But *life sucked balls*. This was my dream . . . but I looked like crap and felt like crap and couldn't taste or smell anything and I couldn't hear and wore that stupid wig and sweated all the time and had been totally betrayed by the body that I talked about long and lovingly in *The Fat Girl's Guide*. It made me feel so sad and frustrated, so compromised. Nothing would be made right for so very long. Even after I got better, there would be so much repair work to do: fixing my nose, finding hearing aids, dealing with cataracts in my eyes, getting rid of the mastoiditis, growing my hair in, getting my body back; all insurmountable . . .

Wait. Why did this litany, easily titled "Things That Are Wrong with Me," sound so familiar? I recognized that voice. Ah yes, it was the Mean Girl again! No wonder her tone was so familiar. Her mockery hadn't started with the autoimmune stuff; it had begun years earlier, the first time my prepubescent tummy muffin-topped my Esprit capris. "You shouldn't look like this," the Mean Girl voice had whispered to me, all the way back in junior high. "You don't love yourself enough. You aren't trying hard enough to change. You don't have it in you. Don't even bother."

I had to shut that beeyotch up. To get healthy in the post-

Cytoxan days, I'd have to change. Live a quiet life. No more crazy work with crazy people. No more middle-of-the-night rice pudding runs on the Lower East Side. I could do it. I made myself a new list, titled "Some Things I Can Do to Feel Better":

*breathe*
*cry*
*stretch, take a walk*
*talk to people I love*
*pray*
*wake up and go to bed at the same time each day*
*take supplements*
*get a massage*
*practice Ayurveda*
*eat fruits and veggies*
*drink tea*
*stay positive*
*make the decision to be here now*
*love/forgive myself*
*let go*

Those sounded suspiciously like suggestions that alternative healers would offer. The spiritualists and the Mean Girl were both motivating me to change.

During a routine CT scan of my chest the following week, a smidge of my abdomen got in the way. The radiologist was concerned about a funky spot in one of the lobes of my liver. The spot wasn't malignant, but the cause was indeterminate. Could be Wegener's, or sarcoidosis, an autoimmune disease similar to Wegener's that usually affects the skin. Could be an abscess, an infection, or a blood clot. Maybe even hepatitis. I wasn't worried about hep; I had none of the risk factors. Turner sent me to a liver specialist, who told me that the problem was probably too much fat in my liver (a syndrome cleverly called "fatty liver") and told me to go on a diet. Always about weight with these guys, isn't it?

I found a different hepatologist, who decided to biopsy my liver in what I now call "My Back Alley Biopsy." Looking back, my guess is that the doc needed some rehearsal poking around, or that a new radiologist wanted to get some diagnostic practice time in on me. I was told to come to the hospital after hours. I didn't bring anyone. I was simply directed to put on a gown and hop up on a table. The doctor explained that he and his team were going to use an ultrasound device to find the appropriate spot, and then guide a long needle into my liver that would scrape out a tiny sample of tissue. I imagined thumb-sized slices of the finest prosciutto (not that I know much about prosciutto; I frequently confuse it with pancetta). The biopsy needle looked like a very slender skewer. Maybe we could use it post-op to make kebabs. A pathologist posted in the room with a microscope would make slides the second they pulled the tissue out, ready to tell us if anything appeared awry. The microscope reminded me of the ones I used to dissect frogs in ninth-grade biology.

The doctor swabbed my abdomen with iodine and shot an

anesthetic into my skin, explaining that he could numb the surface area but had no way to numb the internal organs.

"So, this is going to hurt." I didn't ask, just made a statement.

"Yes, you'll feel the needle go into your liver, but only
once—in an extreme situation, maybe twice—and it will happen
so quickly that you'll barely even notice it."

I felt like I had gone to Thailand for dirt-cheap plastic surgery. I rationalized that I could hack the pain—my pain tolerance
was so high, right? Plus I told myself it would be immediately
beneficial to have an answer right away from the pathologist
who was right in the room. But something didn't smell right, and
not just because I couldn't smell. When I had my original nasal
biopsy, it had been a whole big to-do with early morning hospital arrivals and blood tests, operating theaters and anesthesia.
A whole lot of drama, for what? Now I wanted the drama, more
drama, please, and can I get some of that time-consuming, confusing drama on the side instead of a potentially excruciating,
instant skewering?

I take an enormous amount of pride in my ability to withstand
pain. Once, during eye surgery to repair a tear duct that had been
Weg-enated, the anesthesia didn't take all the way, and I roused.
I was aware of the surgeon scraping something in my face—I
could hear tool on bone—and struggled to get away from him. He
scolded me, "Hey! Stop moving around!" When I saw him at the
surgical follow-up, I asked, "Did you actually have the nerve to
yell at me while I was on the table during surgery?"

"Yeah," he said defending himself. "You were moving around.
It could have screwed me up."

"But I was unconscious!" I protested. "I wasn't responsible for my actions."

"I know," he admitted. "It was just really surprising to me. I always thought of you as such a cool customer."

Note to self, I thought during that consult. Stop being such a cool customer when it comes to pain.

Now I lay on a cot and tried to get into a Zen state of mind. Count my breaths in and out. I was going to have to take in a big breath and hold it once they stuck the needle in there and did their scrape/swab dealio. They rubbed the ultrasound wand on my abdomen and marked a spot. They placed the tip of the kebab thing on the site and told me, "Suck it in and hold it." Then, *pain.*

What does it feel like to have a foot-long needle puncture your skin, push through layers of fat and muscle, clamp on to your liver, scrape out a little chunk, and then pull back out the way it came in? I could almost hear it plunge its way through. It felt like a hot poker—a slender hot poker, but a poker nonetheless, going *charge*! Like the doc was a medieval knight and he just found a soft spot in my armor. Never should have lifted up my arm to wave hello!

There was a pause when he hit the target. I had the smallest beat of "Oh, as long as nothing moves I can handle thi—" and then it pulled back out again. The urge to twist away from it was having a battle royale with my common sense, telling me it would only get worse if I breathed or moved. Out out, dark poker! The doctor and his assistant swung the tip of the needle over to the pathologist, who took a sample to make a slide; they then told me I could breathe again while they had a little consult.

Instant adrenaline-boosted sweat covered my body. Okay, that was bad. That was a 10 on the pain scale. No, more like a 9, because if the needle had been wider it would have caused more pain. For example, a sword wound would be a 10. An average knight on horseback blade was what, a couple of inches wide? This skewer was only a few millimeters in diameter. A 9, then. Not fun, but fast . . . My composure reconstituted itself as the medical experts whispered to each other across the room. The doctor turned back to me with an "Eek, guess what?" bared-tooth smile on his face. "So, here's the thing. We didn't really get enough tissue to read an accurate sample. We're going to have to do it again. I think I told you that it's not unheard-of to have to do this twice."

Oh, God. Again? Not good. But I was already on the table, and swabbed, and at least this time I knew what to expect, and I did want them to get the best sample possible. I vaguely wondered if these were real doctors, or if Harold and Kumar had sneaked in and were pretending to do the job. I gave them a nod of assent and began to breathe in and out as they prepped the wand for round two.

Let me take back what I said before. The thing with the poker being a 9? I'm going to dial it down to an 8, maybe an 8.5, because the first one was way easy compared to round two. I don't know if my body had organized a quick protest and flooded my abdomen with pain-sensitive conscientious objectors, or if the guy didn't shove it in as cleanly the second time, but the first one was distinctly less dramatic than the second. Well, at least I was done.

But of course, I wasn't. The sample still wasn't right. The doctor nervously explained, "The liver is a tricky organ, because it's so big and if you read the wrong part . . ." During round three I gave in to silent tears rolling down my face. I kicked it up a notch for round four, adding a low moan and heavy breathing to the tears. I protested plunge number five, but they swore it was really the very, very last time they would have to do it, and then it would be all over. I rolled on my side and scraped my hands up and down the wall before they could hold me back down. It was after that thrust that I screamed like the first chick to die in a horror movie, having been stabbed repeatedly by a serial killer in a white coat with a mortally ineffective tool. I lurched off the table and out of the room. Only a tiny puncture wound below my breast and a little bit of bruising are proof that My Back Alley Biopsy ever happened.

It wasn't hepatitis A, B, or C. It certainly wasn't fatty liver. The official pathology report came back with inconclusive results: "An unspecified disorder of the liver." My version of a total eclipse of the heart.

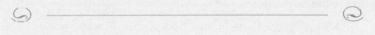

MAY 2004

I threw myself a massive book party at Manhattan's City Bakery, famous for its hot chocolate and pretzel croissants. My goal was to have so much food available for the almost two hundred guests that they'd never think there wasn't more coming: savory apps, tons of sweets, little ramekins of mac-and-cheese. I decided not to wear my wig (which I now regret; those pictures are awful). The night after the party I started a new treatment plan with a drug called Rituxan. Turner explained that it was an off-label prescription for Wegener's but had been successful in treating lymphoma and rheumatoid arthritis. It was a different type of chemotherapeutic regimen. Instead of bombing the whole system, getting rid of the bad stuff along with the good, Rituxan tried to interrupt the message the body gave to immune cells to attack. The treatment involved four weekly infusions at the hospital that took about half a day each. The infusions were pretty similar to what you see on TV or in movies: You go in, hunker down in a La-Z-Boy chair, get hooked up to an IV on a pole, and roll the pole around with you when you go to the bathroom or want to grab a mini-can of ginger ale from the fridge. Most patients brought family or watched TV; I preferred to be on my own. I brought a stack of papers and magazines and would usually pass out half an hour into it, woozy on Benadryl. Rituxan made me feel tired, but it was certainly easier on my system than the oral Cytoxan had been, and presented lower risks in terms of fertility and secondary cancers.

From party to IV pole and back again: Macy's sponsored a national book tour where I'd travel from store to store and host plus-size fashion shows, then sign books. They outfitted me in a thousand dollars' worth of stylish size 22–24 seasonal wardrobe. The best shows were raucous and fun, reminding me that plenty of American women felt quite comfortable showing off their curvy bodies, as long as they had the right outfits to do it in. I sold out of books every time. I was in front of audiences, talking about fashion and body image and making them laugh. Dream come true. But what I mostly remember is going back to the hotel room after the events and crashing into bed, partly from drugs but mostly from exhaustion.

When my headaches got insane, I stayed in full-on Western medical mode and went to a pain clinic at a hospital. It was awful. The most tragic waiting room ever, full of people moaning and one lady screaming in pain. My heart broke for them. A palliative care doctor prescribed a regiment of meds including Trazodone, Topamax, Effexor, Roxicodone, and Kadian, which, doped me into, full slug mode (I assumed he was taking a few himself to cope with the histrionics in the waiting room). Note: watch out for x's in drug names. Those are the naughty ones. Unfortunately, the meds barely dulled the pain. So the doc advised me to take more, and suggested Xanax (double x!) if I needed help sleeping. Not quite. For the first time in my life, I was sleeping like a rock.

Madonna said that she never got into drugs or drinking because she didn't like to lose control. I felt like my life had gone off the rails. I didn't like floating around in a drug fog. I'd rather be in pain and connected to my life than drugged-out and mildly conscious. When I weaned off the drugs and woke up from my semicoma, I decided the Western road had come to an end. Enough with all these doctors, drugs, and pills. I would stay on the essential meds Turner prescribed and keep seeing an ENT, but the poke-'n'-prod era had ended. Time to try something else. I was going to love myself, if not to health, then to death.

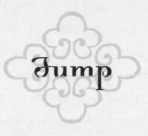

# 9

## Jump

JULY 2004

oly *Viparita Karani*! I found a sweet little Anusara
yoga studio near my apartment and began to practice restorative yoga to get my body moving, even it
was just in the gentlest way. Deb tracked down a female trainer
who came to my apartment and helped me rebuild some strength.
As my exhaustion relented, I started taking walks in the park and
even went back to the gym. It was a major triumph when I lasted
a whole two minutes on the treadmill at a speed of 1.5 miles per
hour. Any issues I'd had about people staring at the fat girl in the
gym totally dissipated. Fuck 'em. I knew victory when I felt it. I'd
won the first heat in the race to self-love. Still, as I rejuvenated,
looking at my crushed nose in the mirror was a constant reminder
that Wegener's ruled my life.

Marta recommended an energy therapist who specialized in
"conscious healing." Beats unconscious healing, I guessed. I went

to her Midtown office in a nondescript building. A pretty, forty-something woman with dark hair welcomed me into the room. I noted a little sitting area, a massage table, and more crystals than I could count. She placed her hands on my body and "read" my energy fields. Her assessment: I had fraught nerve endings, trauma in my system, and grief and sadness in my chest that had to be released. The fourth chakra rides again! We sat and discussed my emotions in an attempt to talk some of the bad energy out of me. I really tried my best to lay it all out there, but it wasn't enough. We had lovely conversations, but she felt more like a friend than a healer. I tried to extend those conversations with a couple of psychotherapists but didn't feel that they could help me tap into the emotional release I needed to get well. Leggo my ego.

Many people in the chronic illness community advised me to try acupuncture. A friend spoke wonders about Frank Lipman, a South African doctor with an office in the Flatiron District. He'd been trained in conventional medicine but preferred to use Eastern modalities and took a holistic approach to health. He had lots of famous clients. I reasoned, If it's good enough for—well, I can't really blow her cover, but you watch her every day on TV—it should be good enough for me.

While Ayurveda was an ancient Indian medical practice that focused on chakras (energy centers) and *prana* (life force) in an attempt to balance *vata, pitta,* and *kapha,* acupuncture is a traditional Chinese medical practice that focuses on meridians (energy channels) and qi (life force) to balance yin and yang. Practitioners insert needles into different meridian points to redirect the qi, improving health and reducing pain. Dr. Lipman had a beautiful, peaceful office and played world music in the waiting room. We had a long consultation before we began any treatment. I found him to be gentle and focused. He was a perfect choice for me because he understood the Wegener's diagnosis from a medical perspective and gave it physiological credence. I liked that he didn't blame me for getting sick. Some other alternative healers either dismissed the concept of autoimmune disease or urged me to stop taking medication. Not an option for me. I couldn't risk it. What I wanted was a treatment that could relieve the worst side effects, complement the meds, and hopefully protect my body from the long-term damage they were causing. Maybe Lipman was the guy who could help me do that.

I'd go into one of the treatment rooms and slip out of my clothes and onto the table, a little gown barely covering me. We'd talk about his practice and my concerns as he delicately pricked needles just under the skin on my torso, legs, ankles, wrists, and even my face. They didn't hurt, but a few really twinged as they went in. This was a good sign, actually, that we were hitting powerful meridian points. Lipman would place earphones on my head filled with the sounds of oceans or chanting, turn down the lights, and leave me to stew for twenty or thirty minutes as I tried to relax. At first I was too worried that I would move and screw up the needles, so I lay frozen on the table like a body in a morgue. But eventually I learned to breathe and tried to use that time each week to check out from the stress of my daily life.

Lipman worked in tandem with a natural pharmacist who prescribed vitamins and supplements and offered dietary guidelines that would relieve inflammation and improve my body's immune function. He backed up every suggestion he made with research, though much of it was still experimental. The acupuncture was expensive, and my insurance company resisted covering it. But it definitely provided relief from the head pain and a window of quiet meditation each week when I had to sit still on that table, slender pins tingling under my skin.

My hunt for nontraditional healing expanded. I went online to find patient-advocacy websites. I hit the alterna-library and read inspiring books by Pema Chödrön, Anne Lamott, and Marianne Williamson. I went to a colonic joint on the Upper West Side. I saw an osteopath who charged me four hundred dollars to tell me I couldn't smell. I moved furniture around in my apartment in a feng shui frenzy, and changed the colors I wore to bring different energy to my body. I placed "charged" crystals around my bed and bathtub. I researched options for stem cell transplants. I went to the Wicca store on Ninth Street in the East Village and had the ladies there whip me up some health potions. I raced around Whole Foods and Whole Body shopping for organic food, soaps, and lotions. Based on recommendations from alternative healers, pals, and online communities, I also tried (in alphabetical order): acidophilus, alpha-lipoic acid, aloe vera gel, arnica, biotin, calcium, coconut oil, CoQ10, glutamine, greens, fermented papaya, fatty fish oil, ginger, lavender, Japanese mushrooms, jojoba oil, magnesium, melatonin, Optiflora, psyllium husk, salt baths, seaweed, sesame oil, soy, St.-John's-wort, Tahitian noni, THC tablets, Thisilyn, tinctures, Valerian root, and vitamins A to zinc. I drank shakes made with flaxseed, frozen berries, beets (and I *hate* beets), red chard, red dandelion, spinach, and water. I went on yeast-free diets, dairy-free diets, mercury-free diets, and alkaline diets. Forget about ingesting a simple carb ever again. I began to get deprivation tremors from my former career as a dieter. I was riding the fine line of becoming one of "those" people.

I felt confident in my decision to pursue complementary healing, and I was living a healthier life in general, but still wasn't seeing major improvement in my diagnostics. The loving miracle men and women of alternative healing were certain that one couldn't separate body from spirit. So if the numbers weren't improving, it must be my fault. I simply didn't want to be healthy. The Mean Girl voice of autoimmune guilt giggled and whispered, louder this time: "That's right. You're not trying hard enough to heal." What a waste of human space I was, the sick equivalent of a fat person who is supposed to be on a diet but keeps eating Oreos anyway. For a woman who'd written a book called *The Fat Girl's Guide to Life*, the irony was thicker than hot fudge. I deserved chronic illness. I wasn't maintaining a rigid daily spiritual practice. I hadn't moved to a pasture in the countryside. I still used Sweet'N Low. I spritzed Windex on my counters and laundered my clothes with Tide. I'd been advised to inject spider poison and chew Amazonian jungle bark to make myself healthy, but didn't do it. Why not?

Well, maybe because it sounded crazy. But maybe because I didn't love myself enough. Because I wouldn't let go of my pain. I was to blame for my disease, like a rape victim who'd been wearing a short skirt when she'd been assaulted. Wegener's was the rapist. I was Jodie Foster. A doctor would say that it had nothing to do with me. I didn't ask for Wegener's. But in the private court of alternative medicine, I'm sure some mantra-chanting practitioners meditated to themselves, "Girlfriend wouldn't be in this fix if only she'd worn sweatpants!"

I heard this message over and over: "There's a reason you are suffering. . . . You have been chosen for this, Wendy. . . . This is a lesson you have to learn." Some possible Life 101's from the "Let Go" series: I was moving too fast, living too loose, going off the road. I needed to love, cry, stop and smell the roses (again, couldn't smell!). Clearly, practitioners and healers explained, a sick person had some sort of choice about the situation. My soul was bigger, better, smarter than the limits of modern medicine. They had to be right. There must be more I could do to help myself live, and live well. Instead of wasting time reading *Entertainment Weekly* and watching *Arrested Development*, I had to look inside myself, light candles, and chant my mantra. I could be one downward dog away from undoing the damage that had gotten me sick in the first place! I needed to go deeper, release myself from negative emotions like fear and anger that had turned my body against me. Go back through my life and forgive, as Rai had advised.

This concept of having a choice about illness was a new one for me. I didn't understand that you could live with illness, that there could be some sort of middle ground. My experience after losing my mom was that one day you were fine and the next day you were gone. Alive or dead. Feel perfectly fine or plan a funeral. The in-between—tests, waiting, doctor's appointments, medications, side effects, fear, and relief—was uncharted territory for me.

So I had to MapQuest a road to revelation: Look into my heart, dig deep into that fourth chakra, and find my mother. I concluded that the spiritual people were right. If I wanted health, it wasn't going to show up in pill form.

---

NOVEMBER 2004

That Thanksgiving, my friends Pam and Ady invited me to join them at the Kripalu Center for Yoga & Health, a world-famous alternative healing institute in the Berkshires. I needed a break; I'd just finished working on the supercool *Glamour* Women of the Year Awards, crafting speeches for celebs like Susan Sarandon and Katie Couric, and shooting a TV special with Buffy herself, Sarah Michelle Gellar. I was pooped. Kripalu's weekend "rest and relaxation" program would cost around six hundred dollars. Instead of a turkey dinner, we'd be bringing in our day of thanks with bowls of quinoa and kale. Any self-love or enlightenment I could dig up would be just terrif, and I also hoped some expert there could help me break a record eighteen-day constipation fest.

Originally built as a Jesuit seminary, Kripalu retained a dormitory feel. When all the shoes were stacked outside conference rooms where clients did yoga and meditation, mine were the only glittery slip-on Skechers in the bunch (at least I knew to bring slip-ons this time). The staff requested that we avoid using soap and shampoos, so that our scent wouldn't throw off anyone else in yoga classes. Didn't bother me; I couldn't smell a thing. Plus my digestive tract was so packed with crap that I could barely bend over in *Uttanasana* pose. I felt like a casing packed with shit. A shit sausage. On Thanksgiving Day, as we took a walk in the snow-covered woods (Pam and Ady walked; it's more like I lumbered), I recalled the events of a year earlier, when I'd gone to the hospital and the Cytoxan saga had begun. I'd been so down physically and mentally, then tried so hard to turn it around, even if there was that annoying part of me that didn't want to get better. Why wouldn't I?

Pam and Ady highly recommended a session with Prama, their energy healer and massage therapist at Kripalu. Pam was one of my most rational friends; I figured if she trusted her body to Prama, she had to be good. Halfway through day nineteen of my nonpoopage marathon, the two of us sat in her small, calm office and talked before I got up on her table. Prama had clean-energy beauty, and a peaceful demeanor. On the surface Prama could be considered a Gray Braider, but I was trying not to be so judgmental about appearances anymore. I had a feeling she wasn't named "Prama" from the git-go. Maybe like . . . Susan Rosenthal or something? Like spiritual teacher Ram Dass, who had been born nice Jewish boy Richard Alpert. I wondered what moved her to be a healer, if she'd had a personal crisis in her own life that led her down this road. Kripalu had just started offering a *panchakarma* program (Rai even taught classes there), and it helped me to describe my medical history to Prama in Western and Ayurvedic terms. I wrapped up my story with, "So I'm still on all of this medication and I can't take a dump. I don't know if I should be doing Western or Eastern. If I go Eastern, should it be Ayurveda or Chinese medicine? If I do Ayurveda, do I have to move to New Mexico? I can't even believe I'm asking some of these questions. When I hear myself, I think, Uch, I sound so goofy and New Age." Prama gave a gentle laugh. I concluded, "I'm trying as hard as I can but I can't seem to get out of this . . . funk. I'm worried that there's a part of me that doesn't want to get better. But that makes no sense."

Prama explained, "This sounds like an issue of *pitta* versus *kapha*. You were doing this crazy job, living this crazy life—a *pitta* life, to an extreme. Now, this sickness is like a big, cold, wet blanket put on you. That blanket is *kapha*. Your unwillingness to shift out of that *kapha* state could be your system telling you, 'I don't want to go back to that extreme *pitta* place.' But *you don't have to.*

"There is a place in between the two. It already exists. You need to work to find this middle space. Life doesn't always have to be like this . . ." Prama made a big wavy motion with her arm. It was a sine wave, or a cosine wave. I could never get it straight in algebra class. "Sometimes it can be like this." She made the same wave, but much slower, with the highs and lows much smaller. Prama continued: "So when you have a question or concern about your health, about 'What do I do next?' that can be answered with: 'What's in the middle?' It doesn't have to be full *panchakarma* or nothing. It can be one *abhyanga* massage. You worry about failing; you ask yourself, 'What did I learn?' You worry about doing Ayurveda versus doing Chinese medicine so you do neither. It doesn't matter which one you do. You worry that you're going to seem 'goofy' or 'New Age'? Get over your arrogance."

Busted. It hadn't occurred to me that my derision of all things foo-foo was arrogant. But it was. It was a certain brand of Manhattan city mouse snobbery, like looking down on hair mousse or Brooklyn. She was right, though. Who was I to judge what way people chose to make themselves feel better? If it was therapy and Valium, fine. If it was green tea and dreadlocks, so be it.

"I believe what you're going through . . . this process has purpose," Prama explained gently. "Maybe it's to help yourself. Maybe it's to help others. Maybe you'll write about it someday." I'd heard this theory a million times. It always felt like a reach. The situation was what it was. I laughed and said, "It better have purpose. It would sure be a waste to go through this for nothing."

She looked me in the eye, unwilling to let me use a joke as a defense mechanism. "Keep searching for the middle place. It doesn't have to be all sleep or no sleep. Take a fifteen-minute power nap. You don't have to be rigid or in a free fall. Make a schedule, but build into it blocks of free time. And you just won't know what you'll do with them till you're there. This is the battle, between yin and yang, right and left, masculine and feminine. The left side of the body is masculine but the right side is feminine. The left side of the mind is rational; the right side is creative. So use both. Make creative, rational decisions. Try to find the wise mind in the middle."

When would I ever get this through my granuloma-ridden

skull, that things didn't have to be black or white? Gray was okay. I lived my life as fat or thin. Healthy or sick. Light or dark. I never even considered the middle to be an option. I had to get my "maybe" on. Maybe Prama was the guru I'd been looking for all this time.

That evening during Sharing Circle (theme: "The Possibility of Gratitude"), I raced back to the bathroom in our hall and ended my constipation marathon. Even without PK, Prama had given me an emotional *basti.* I planned to embrace her advice and try to find "the wise mind in the middle."

When I returned to the city, I caught up on the stack of the previous week's *New York Times* sitting outside my apartment door. I read a story about a young woman who decided to throw a party by following the advice of Dorothy Draper, a famous hostess and interior designer in the 1940s and '50s. The writer said:

> Dorothy Draper changed my mind, in part by convincing me that being a good hostess is a matter of attitude. She urges party givers to distinguish between "the inner YOU," which might be "shy, sensitive, and easily hurt," and "the outer YOU," which is seen by "your mirror, your hairdresser, your family and the friends who know you so well that they don't mince matters." She suggests that all the hostess needs to do to bridge this gap is to

"make friends with yourself" and above all avoid the
"Will to Be Dreary," the woeful state of "being resigned
to life and terribly serious about it."*

Bridging the gap. Making friends with myself. It was the missing link to finding my way to the middle where I could love myself
correctly and get healthy again. I couldn't dwell on ambivalence.
Ambivalence sucks, as dreary as it gets. I would banish the will to
be dreary.

 ────────────────────────────────

### DECEMBER 6, 2004

### MY 33RD BIRTHDAY

**CURRENT FAVORITE MOVIE:**
*Wanted to love* The Life Aquatic with Steve Zissou;
*now I think Wes Anderson must be kidding (but Seu
Jorge's Portuguese Bowie covers are brill)*

**CURRENT FAVORITE TV SHOW:**
*Loving* Lost. *My theory: It's a take on* The Wizard of
Oz *(Kate = Dorothy, Jack = Scarecrow, Sawyer = Tin
Man, Hurley = Cowardly Lion, Locke = Wizard)*

**CURRENT CRAZY LADY:**
*Lindsay Lohan. She was such a cutie when I worked with
her at MTV; what the hell happened? Acoustically
challenged Ashlee Simpson on her tail*

---

* Eva Hagberg, "Hostess With the Mostes' Jitters," *New York Times*, November 18,
2004.

IN MADONNA NEWS:
*British tabloids report that while shooting an ad campaign
for Versace, Madonna fired her manager for not adhering
to the tenets of Kabbalah*

O n my thirty-third birthday, my friend Kimmi told me that
33 = 3 + 3 = 6, which is the lovers' card in tarot. "It's
more than just the kind of love you feel while you're wearing
panties and a slip," she said, it's also "the struggle of the two sides
of the self to work together, and find balance." That resonated. I
looked in the mirror and noticed . . . the bob was back! My hair
was growing in. I could almost see myself again. I made an appointment with Dorothy, who trimmed and shaped it. We both
smiled into her mirror at the end of the cut. "I have so much
power," she nodded, approving of the transformation.

I focused on the intention of finding balance, trying to pray
for peace and health for myself. I hoped I had purpose. Even if I
wasn't sure what that purpose was, it had to be worth finding. I
felt like I'd been knocked out by this huge challenge but was
starting to stir on the mat. My Wegener's symptoms began to
improve. My thirty-third birthday left only two years on my Life
Clock, but maybe there was a chance I'd still beat it. If Gwyneth
could drop out of the movie business to raise daughter Apple,
I could make big changes, too. I could try harder, and this time I
would succeed.

I redoubled my efforts to meditate. Everyone who was healthy
said it was essential, and even if I didn't do it for a long time, at
least I could do something. Kind of like working out. Come on,

twenty minutes a day? Not too much to ask. But there were days that I skipped. Emmy and I went to a Shakti Gawain seminar in L.A. to practice "creative visualization." It wasn't difficult to visualize a giant pink ball of love descending on me, but I felt (shh) kinda silly. As a measure of good faith I carried Shakti's book around with me everywhere I went, so that self-awareness might seep into me by osmosis. Kind of like Britney schlepping around Kabbalah books as she strutted in and out of Starbucks. I did *pranayama* breathing exercises in Riverside Park, trying to see the beauty in rotten people and stay really connected and focused . . . but sometimes I just wanted to eat banana cake and watch TV. I followed Andrew Weil's *Spontaneous Healing* eating plan, very sensible as I loved salmon, legumes, and blueberries, but every once in a while a girl needs a Diet Coke with lemon! I'm sorry but it's true!

Technically that sounds like balance. In my head, I can see that it was. But in my heart it always feels like I'm excelling at bad behavior while the good stuff has a long way to go. Finding the middle isn't as easy as it looks.

m y hearing began to fade as the teeny bones in my inner ears melted into Wegener-related mush. My ENT described it to me as if I'd had a fire in my head. Even though the fire was out, the embers were still smoldering. I had to get hearing aids in both ears ($3,500 each, with no insurance coverage, thank you very much). I completely lost my sense of smell as my olfactory nerves wore away. Doctors said it wouldn't come back. It's easy for people to comprehend hearing loss, but smelling loss is harder to describe. At first everything smelled awful, chemical, then like rot. Then for a while I could tell there was a smell, but I just couldn't identify what it was. Then, nothing.

This "anosmia," aka ass-nosmia, was not necessarily a curse. I could go into a public bathroom almost anywhere in the world (Target, Yankee Stadium, gas station john that Britney has recently visited sans shoes) without being fazed. Upstairs neighbor cooking teriyaki stir-fry again? Residue of homeless guy who relieved himself on the corner of Forty-fourth and Broadway in the middle of August? Mysterious maple syrup smell that wafted over New York and turned out to be a New Jersey factory using fenugreek to make food fragrances?* Not issues for me.

Nary an odor irked me at the gym, whether it was funky towels or stuffy showers; the entire locker room genre was no problem. Once, I took the World's Most Terrible Yoga Class at my gym. (Sidebar: Automatically a no-no. Do not take yoga at a gym. It's like buying groceries at a drugstore. Any so-called nutrition you can buy at a Walgreen's can't be good for you.) Anyway, I thought the class sucked because our mats were pointed into the center of the room and the teacher wandered around touching people instead of demonstrating the positions. I was stuck right under a speaker and a clock. I couldn't hear a word of his instruction

---

* "The strange, syrupy scent has descended on parts of New York City and New Jersey at least three times before. . . . Some have theorized that the smell came from New Jersey." Trymaine Lee, "Mysterious Sweet Smell from 2005 Returns to Manhattan," *New York Times*, January 6, 2009.

because he seemed to think that blasting Chaka Khan and Joy Division would make for ideal yoga accompaniment music. He saw me looking around at the other students for some sort of clue, and said, "Don't worry about what everyone else is doing. Just do what feels right to you." Well, what feels right to me is staying home and watching reruns of *The Colbert Report*, so that's not gonna be a winning strategy, Swami Boy. He sauntered around telling stories and interrupting himself to make a horrible noise that sounded like "*eeeeeccchhhhhh,*" which I now believe was his interpretation of deep *ujjayi* breathing. So we were getting a sound track of:

*"I was once at this flea market with my guru and EEEEECCCHHHHHH"*

CHAKA EVERYBODY
EVERYBODY CHAKA KHAN

*". . . he was completely mystical in the way he looked at a bunch of old car parts EEEEECCCHHHHHH"*

I FEEL FOR YOU,
I THINK I LOVE YOU

*"Don't worry about what everyone else is doing EEEEECCCHHHHHH"*

*(harmonica solo)*

He only stopped wandering and chatting to say, "It smells like sewage down at that end of the studio. Especially the people under the clock. Wow, I feel bad for you *eeeeeccchhhhhh*." I was so grateful my nose didn't work. If I'd known that in addition to everything else I was downward dogging in a stew of stink, I would have punched the guy.

But without a complete olfactory system I missed out on a lot of good stuff, obvious winners, like the scents of freesia and garlic bread. The upside was that my emotional appetite was never tripped off by a breadbasket. I didn't get hungry at street fairs or crave those nuts they sell on New York City streets at Christmas. I made an excellent babysitter for little kids because changing diapers didn't bug me a bit. Then again, I couldn't tell when they needed their diapers changed unless I took a peek or a poke.

The situation presented certain technical problems. For example, postexercise, could I get away with running errands or was I all BO-ey? Was the sweater I'd worn three days in a row clean or dirty? There was nothing I wouldn't Febreze. I didn't even know what Febreze smelled like. I assumed it was like a breeze in February, whatever that might be . . . fresh and crisp? I hoped it was working. (When I have a trusted friend over, I go through a stack of clothes and do a smell test. You've got to really care about someone to get up and personal with the nubs on a pal's underwire in the armpit.)

Farting. I no longer knew with certainty if I did or not, so I erred on the side of "wave it out of there." I hadn't lit a match in the bathroom for years but I could change if I had someone living with me.

I did a long stint washing my hair with potent Indian Ayurvedic shampoos without realizing that people were passing out from my overwhelming sandalwood and sesame oil scent. When eating bagels, I never knew if I got all of the tuna fish or lox off my hands, or the peanut butter. I didn't know when I stepped in dog shit and tracked it into someone's house (please, neighbors, make an effort to clean up after your French bulldogs and pugs). Did my perfume make me smell alluring or hooker-iffic? Was someone smoking weed at my party? I had no idea. You'd be surprised how many times people say, "Can you smell that?" or "How good does that smell?" I'd just nod along and fake it ("Hmm, yeah!"), because it takes a while to explain to someone that I really can't smell anything. I made the mistake of telling my friend's four-year-old about it and every time I saw her she'd test me. "Can you smell *that*? But can you smell *that*?"

Smell-lessness was dangerous in ways I'd never thought about. There was no warning signal when the milk went bad, since I couldn't sniff out sour. That meant I had to buy milk almost every day or else I ended up doing some pretty nasty taste tests. One day Josh opened my refrigerator and took a whiff. "Something is rotting in here!" Can you at least tell me what it is? Was the garbage stinky? Was whatever was in the oven ready (as if there were ever anything in the oven)? If the gas were on, would I smell it? What if there were a fire and I couldn't smell smoke? I was the human equivalent of a fire detector with a dead battery in it. As it turned out, there was once a gas leak in my apartment building. I only noticed when I cranked up my hearing aids and heard the sound of sirens on my street. Firemen stormed the building and banged on my door. "Do you smell gas in there?" they shouted. The look on their faces as I tried to explain that no I didn't, but there could be gas floating around, because I had no sense of smell . . . I probably came off like one of the crazier locals.

It wasn't like my other senses became keener after I lost my sense of smell. I didn't see better because I couldn't smell. I'd be the lamest vampire in history. But if I had to give up a sense voluntarily, smell would be the first one to go. I'd rather be smell-less than blind or deaf (even though I was on my way there, too). Think about Beethoven. There he was, almost completely sound-proofed, forging ahead and writing those symphonies. Can you say, "bitter"? I was sad about my smell deficiencies, but it wasn't like I was a perfumer for a living. He was the world's greatest composer. He lost his sense of hearing. That's an awful fate. My friend Meghan told me that Michael Hutchence, the lead singer of INXS, killed himself because he couldn't smell (not just a general nonsmell, but particularly, ahem, the scent of a woman). I thought he'd choked himself accidentally through autoerotic asphyxiation. Either way, not a happy ending.

It would suck if I couldn't touch anything, if I had absolutely no tactile sense. I wasn't sure if it was physically possible, although they seemed to have an article every year or two in *People* magazine about kids with some rare genetic disorder who kept putting their fingers in hot pans because they couldn't feel pain. (Even if they couldn't sense pain, you'd think someone would tell them not to touch glowing red pans on stoves.)

Luckily, my sense of taste had remained secure, as the taste buds on my tongue were different than the olfactory patch high up in my nose that had worn away. I definitely enjoyed spicier things but my palate was the same as ever; that is, I had yet to see anyone on *Top Chef* make anything that I wanted to eat.

But there's more to just smell than simply scent. Smell triggers emotional recall. Things you can't describe, such as the smell of the airport in Miami or the house you grew up in. The individual odors of the people you love. I remember the spicy, roasted smell of my grandpa Mark's tobacco, but I won't ever be able to get another hit of it. You know how animals can track prey or find family members by getting a whiff of them? I couldn't. If I were an emperor penguin chick doing that mating march I'd be screwed. Without the ability to sniff out my family's individual breeding ground, I'd be left on an arctic beach all by myself and a leopard seal would maul me. If I were stuck on the island in *Lost* I'd never be able to point my nose in the air and say, "Sawyer, the ocean's thataway!" Again, I encourage anyone nearby during a disaster to squelch the life out of me and eat me first.

Then there was the whole pheromone issue, the hormone-based odor that humans give off to signify sexual availability or attraction. If that were the way I'd fall in love with someone, but I couldn't smell him, would I ever fall in love? There was that infamous study about what smells arouse men the most—the winners were pumpkin pie, doughnuts, and lavender.* I'd have to lurk around a Dunkin' Donuts to meet my soulmate.

I made a list (I often do):

SMELLS I MISS

*Nail salons*
*Fall, that crispy smell on the first cold night*
*Bounce*
*Bactine*
*The stink in my hair after a long night out* (restaurant & bar &
  perfume & boy & alcohol & cigarettes, back in the day)
*Jennifer Lopez* (she wafted past me at a *Glamour* magazine
  event one year and smelled like everything good all at
  once—toasty bread and butter with cinnamon and
  perfume and beach)
*Baby shampoo*
*Chlorine*
*Franklin Cider Mill doughnuts*
*Our house in Michigan when I go home on vacation*
*Softsoap hand soap*

---

* "Pumpkin pie and lavender, and other food smells like doughnuts and licorice . . . were the most sexually tantalizing of those tested in a study carried out in the late 1990s by Dr. Alan R. Hirsch, who directs the Smell and Taste Treatment and Research Foundation in Chicago." Scott McCredie, "Aroma and Arousal," MSN Health & Fitness.

*Hair dye*

*Opium perfume*

*Our dog Inky* (but he's dead so that doesn't count; I can't
    smell him anyway)

*Coffee* (if only Starbucks smelled awesome)

*Celestial Seasonings Roastaroma tea*

*Wire hanger smell on your hands after you handle one*

*Permanent marker ink*

*Jergens lotion*

## SMELLS I DON'T MISS

*New York streets in the summertime*

*Baby aspirin*

*Drakkar Noir cologne* (Why they sent the memo out to guys
    in the '80s that they all had to wear it, I'll never know)

*Things that are supposed to smell "orange"*

*Dirty sponges*

*Commercial mops, the stringy kind, especially when they've
    been used a lot*

*Ice-cream parlors*

## SMELLS I COULD CARE LESS ABOUT (THAT OTHER PEOPLE LIKE HATE)

*Baby powder*

*Roses*

*Freshly cut grass*

*BBQ*

*Dirty socks*

*Bonfires*

*New car* (So what? Completely overrated)

The Sanskrit word for breath is *prana*. To the yogic folks, *prana* is more than air; it's really a life or energy force (also known in other modalities as chi or qi). When we sniff and breathe, we intake and output *prana*. *Prana* is everywhere. At the Ayurvedic Center and yoga classes, we were taught *pranayama* breathing exercises. A teacher once told me that "the pole of *prana*" began eight finger breadths away from my nose. If I stacked eight fingers away from my nose, that would be the area where I should aim to breathe the *prana* in. But if my nose didn't work properly, and the channels to breathe in scents and air and *prana* were blocked, and *prana* was life force, I worried: Did I have no life? At least I had one sign of hope; when I sliced onions, I still cried.

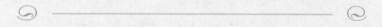

MARCH 2005

The following spring I went back to see Dr. Rai for a third week of *panchakarma* detox, by myself this time. No distractions. I closed my eyes as he gave the class my diagnosis. My attitudes and habits were dramatically different since my last trip to New Mexico. I'd been working as hard as I could to find balance and forgive. My *vikruti* would certainly reflect that. For the third time, he gently meditated while listening to my pulse, then announced, "*Vata*, one; *pitta*, three-point-five; *kapha* . . . three-point-five. Maybe four."

My eyes snapped open as I sputtered, "But that's even worse than last time!"

He gave me a sympathetic look that was becoming all too familiar. "No better, no worse, Shan-kar. Just what is."

I was so frustrated that my chromatherapy session was a nonstarter. Michael, the facilitator, told me, "Your energy is cutting off your heart and moving everything to your brain." I bristled through my final meeting with Rai, glaring at his ridiculous elephant decorations and his stupid tree friend. He paused and looked at me. "You are a very beautiful person, Shan-kar. You have beautiful thoughts. But this expectation . . ." He sighed. "You must love yourself as you are."

Love myself as I am? Irate, I stomped back through the soccer field to herby, smelly, stinky Lotus House. I'd been through this kind of frustration when I was trying to lose weight. Worked so hard, thought I excelled, and then . . . no results. Life, health, wellness . . . whatever you call it, my search for balance felt just like dieting, when I berated myself with every failure that if I had only tried harder, I would have lost the weight.

When I got to the soccer goal, I stopped. Hold up. Hadn't I realized that the weight blame game was bullshit? I was no more to blame for being sick than I was for being fat. I kept looking for a wellness epiphany that would fix me, just as dieters long for a "magic pill" to pop that will make them thin and happy. I kept bouncing between Ayurveda, acupuncture, supplements, yoga—like signing up for Weight Watchers, Jenny Craig, personal trainer—sure that this practice was the right practice. It worked for so many other people! If it didn't work for me, it had to be because I wasn't trying hard enough.

Rai once explained to his students in front of me, "People with 'autoimmune diseases' do not love themselves." That also rang an old bell. If I loved myself enough, I'd make myself thin. Now, if I loved myself enough, I'd make myself well. That was simply not the case. Having a positive attitude might give me an edge, but there was no one-to-one ratio between self-love and health. Do people who love themselves a lot stay healthier than people who love themselves a little? No. Do all healthy people adore themselves, or are some full of both vitality and self-hate? Yes. Does every sick person loathe herself? No. Do people who have on-and-off self-love affairs only get minor diseases, like colds? No.

I got Wegener's *because I got Wegener's.* I have issues of grief and anger. Sure nuff. I find it next to impossible to live a toxin-free life. Okay. But why I got it—why anyone gets any illness—is pretty much a crapshoot. There are factors of causation, like genetics or high-risk living, or owning a trailer home in Chernobyl. There are lifelong smokers who die of old age and squeaky-clean triathletes who die of lung cancer. There are alcoholics who drink themselves silly without a peep from their livers, and children who die of hepatitis. There are innocent, loving, forgiving people who die horrible, violent deaths, and Nazi war criminals who die peacefully on the beach in Brazil. Call it karma, fate, bad luck, happenstance. It's not fair, but it's certainly not an issue of fault.

So I would try my very best to be healthy. But I'd do it on my terms, following protocols that made sense for my life. There is clearly some correlation between happiness, positivity, and clean living, but it's not necessarily a "vibe" thing. All of those qualities lower stress, at least in my body. Lower stress means less surging cortisol, means happier Wendy. My revised plan: a little medicine, a little meditation. A little surgery, a little seaweed. Some folic acid and some forgiveness. In other words, a healthy balance between two forces.

If that ain't the wise mind in the middle, I don't know what is.

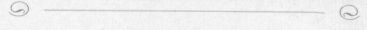

APRIL 2005

The best intentions still don't ensure the best outcome. A month after my trip to New Mexico I woke up in horrible pain, every joint screaming. I was basically immobilized with pain. Even Oxycodone, which had recently given me some measure of relief, didn't help. I panicked. I'd spent months putting together deals with networks including Lifetime and ABC to turn my book into a reality show. The meeting to sign the paperwork was at 4 p.m. How was I possibly going to make it to a meeting, and also muster up the energy to be my most fabulous self? Luckily Myrn was in town. She came to my place, put clothes and jewelry on me, did my hair and makeup. I still could not lift my arms, could not move. I called my agent and told him to cancel the meeting. He told me that unless I came in and signed the papers, the deal would fall off the table. I said, "Screw it." Screw everything. The deal. The career. My life. I already knew: The Wegener's was back in full force.

# 10

# Papa Don't Preach

When I was first diagnosed with Wegener's granulomatosis, I wondered why I couldn't get a Jewish disease. I'm not talking about genetic predisposition; by "Jewish" I mean the tenor of the disease itself. For example, my impression of cystic fibrosis is that it's not a Jewish disease. Not to say that Jews don't get it; it's just not on our radar. But lymphoma? There's a Jewish disease. Mysterious and tragic, and most people don't know exactly what it is. We seem to deal with a lot of cancer, hypothyroidism, and anything that screws up the digestive tract.

Jewish people prefer to go to Jewish doctors. Occasionally we'll make an exception for an Indian guy in an emergency room. But someone named "McSomething" or "Somethingelli" will rarely get near a Jewish organ. It's a ghetto mentality based on the (not altogether) unjustified conviction that everyone wants to see us dead, combined with the deep-seated Jewish belief that somehow we are "chosen" above all others, plus some residual "Are you really going to leave your life in the hands of someone who was WASPy enough to be a cheerleader in high school?" doubt. We thrive on fatalism. I'm one of the few people my age who stashes a Baggie full of silverware that I'm willing to trade for medicine and/or passage out of the country under my bed.

If the Children of Israel are the Chosen Ones, that sometimes makes God feel like our abusive alcoholic daddy figure. He keeps testing us, doing horrible things to us depending on his mood (slavery, hate crimes, concentration camps, inquisitions) and we keep making excuses for Him, telling ourselves that He's only doing it because He loves us, or else He wants us to prove our commitment to Him. At some point we're going to have to get Dr. Drew (a Jew) to stage a holy intervention.

Another Jewish medical prerequisite: We will not confer with anyone less than "the Best Guy." Need a colonoscopy? "I know the Best Guy at Lenox Hill." Heart skipping a beat? "I know a cardiologist, best one in his class at Harvard Medical School." Strange mass on your inner thigh? "I know this dermatologist, best guy in the city, and he'll do a little Botox while you're waiting." (The Best Guy is never a woman. Even gynecologists are always Best Guys.) With Jews occupying all the seats in the best doctors' waiting rooms, and consulting with the best doctors' labs and pathologists, I wonder how people of other faiths can get anything close to quality health care.

We do take great pride in Jewish advances in science and medicine, which admittedly are many. Einstein? A Jew. Salk? A Jew. Freud? A Jew, and look how he changed our perceptions of society. Jewish people will swear that any new successful diagnostic machine was built originally for the Israeli army.

I found it took forever to explain my diagnosis to some of

my fellow Jews. They kept interrupting to mention who they knew who was related to someone who happened to have that exact disease. Then, as we were talking, the Jew across from me would always turn out to know the Best Guy in (rheumatology/otolaryngology/pulmonology/ophthalmology/dermatology), so I'd have to stop and write that down. Plus we instinctively say "God forbid" between every negative thing, in case—God forbid—God should hear me discussing my random disease and decide to punish me for good. Here's a sample conversation:

JEW: What's the disease called?
ME: Wegener's granulomatosis.
JEW: Spell that.
ME: W-E-G-E-N—
JEW: N, E . . . Yeah, yeah, I got it close enough. Wait— You know what? I think my brother's wife's mother has exactly the same thing.
ME: Really?
JEW: Yeah, with the edema [edema, Jewish; emphysema, not Jewish] and the blood clotting and the nerve damage?
ME: Not exactly . . .
JEW: I know the Best Guy! His name is Somethingberg/stein/feld. He went to Harvard Medical School, graduated top of his class, and he happens to be the number one cardiothoracic surgeon in the country.
ME: Um, it's not really heart disease, but I'll try anything at this point.

JEW: Listen: If God forbid this should turn out to be something to worry about God forbid, he can at least tell you what side effects God forbid or what research they are doing if God forbid you should really have this disease. My niece lives in Tel Aviv, so I'll ask her, too. Did you know that Israelis used war technology to invent the standing MRI?

ME: Just because someone lives in Tel Aviv—

JEW: Exactly. We're not going to worry until we know that God forbid there is something to worry about. Bye!

I felt like I had started on the wrong foot: the *goyishe* foot. Why hadn't I called in the Jewish cavalry to tell me who all the Best Guys were? When the whole thing started, I had no idea how many Best Guys would need to get involved.

One way my parents responded to my illness was to turn to God. Even though they were nice Jewish parents who lived in a nice Jewish neighborhood, their current faith was slightly different than the one we grew up with. I was down with God; Mick and Myrn were down with G-DASH-D. When I was in high school, they went from being typical North American Reform Jews who celebrate holidays and send their kids to Jewish summer camps to active members of a Lubavitcher shul.

Lubavitchers are followers of the Orthodox missionary Chabad-Lubavitch movement. The consonants that make up the word *Chabad* in Hebrew stand for Wisdom, Understanding, and Knowledge. Some of these folks are qualified to teach Madonna's spiritual quest of choice, Kabbalah, or Jewish mysticism. The designations of Jewish religious movements (Reform, Conservative, Orthodox, and so on) are more about practice than faith; someone can be a very liberal Jew in practice but have just as much faith as the more Orthodox practitioners on the planet.

One day a Lubavitcher rabbi came to our door to pick up our *pushke*, a little tin box we'd put loose change in to give to charity. My parents invited him in. Next thing I know, Mick is offering to set me up in an arranged marriage.

By nature, Myrn has a devout soul, a healthy collection of superstitions (watch out for the Evil Eye!) and a surprisingly handy collection of Yiddish slang ("This air-conditioning . . . what a *mechiah*!"*). At first she was excited to create a kosher kitchen, where she would follow strict dietary laws that separated milk from meat. Plus it was fun to shop for all new flatware and dishes. But at Chabad services she had to sit with women only, who were raised in a very different tradition. She could certainly relate as a nurturer, but very few of the other women shared her passion for nineteenth-century toile, or had a crush on Anderson Cooper.

Mick started the daily ritual of laying tefillin, a practice where men wrap leather boxes filled with holy scrolls on their arms. It's kind of like meditation, but with cooler props. He also nailed mezuzot (decorative cases for holy scrolls) on every door in the house. Pictures of the Lubavitch movement's leader (Rabbi

---

* "What a relief!"

Schneerson, aka "the Rebbe") joined our family photos on the wall. Though he had died years before, many of Schneerson's followers felt that he was the Messiah.

This shift in religious practices led to some stress in our family. As an ardent feminist, I would hear none of it. As an ardent intellectual, my brother refused. Still, my folks always invited us to join them on their spiritual adventures, like a visit to Rabbi Baumbacher's house to say hi to his sixteen children (including two sets of twins!), or *kapparot*, the ritual sacrifice of chickens on the high holidays (recently condemned by PETA) as symbolic atonement for sin, followed by a charitable donation. I knew we were in deep when eating dinner at the Village Place restaurant in my hometown, I saw my car—*my* car that I was so grateful to receive as a Sweet Sixteen present, the one I drove all through high school and college—my car sailed by with a giant menorah strapped to the roof and a sign that read CHABAD LUBAVITCH OF WEST BLOOMFIELD, MICHIGAN on the door. I recognized the license plate: 835 TUX. "Dad," I sputtered, "I could swear that was my Ford Taurus that just went by!"

"Oh yeah." He smiled. "I gave it to Rabbi Baumbacher. It *was* a Ford Taurus. Now it's a Mitzvah Mobile!"

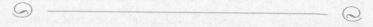

JUNE 2004

mick came to visit me in New York on Father's Day. Earlier that morning I'd had an appointment with Celeste, an intuitive body worker recommended to me by my acupuncturist, Dr. Lipman. It took months to get on her schedule. I was surprised when I walked into the office and saw her; Celeste was the polar opposite of the Gray Braid club. She had delicate features, long blond hair, sexy shoes, and a bangin' designer handbag. When I asked how she got into this line of work, Celeste explained that she had a friend who had gotten cancer, and while caring for her discovered a talent for "reading the body." She didn't charge her clients; she felt that using her ability to heal people was her way of giving back to whatever powers had helped her friend eventually recover.

I climbed up on a table in Lipman's office. For a few minutes, Celeste placed her hands on different parts of my body as I tried to get all Zen in my mind. Then she diagnosed my health problem from her point of view: "You have fear stored in your fourth chakra." Fear? Really? What a refreshing change from grief! "It's surprising, actually, because usually you find fear in the lower chakras."

Celeste continued, "You also have a blockage in the sixth chakra." That was the spot on my forehead between my brows where they dripped the *shirodhara* oils, the same place where I sliced my forehead open. My third eye. Apparently I had a severe case of Third Eye Blind, in addition to the scar from the split up the center of my forehead. "Really, it feels like you have a crazy switch on."

"I'm on a ton of steroids," I explained.

"I'm going to do what I can to turn it off. I'm also going to try to get under the chemo drugs and see if I can open up that blockage." She laid her hands on me again for a few more moments, then grabbed her D&G or Louis Vuitton and headed back home to Connecticut.

madonna was at Madison Square Garden on the Re-Invention tour that night, but I passed up the show to hang out with Mick. I had also skipped the show the night before (on the summer solstice, no less!) for a book reading. At least I knew I was going to a Madonna show later that week with Emmy.

On the way to dinner at a kosher restaurant on the Upper West Side, I explained Celeste's "blockage" theory to Mick. He thought it was utter nonsense but at that point was too concerned about my health to completely dismiss any idea that might work. Suddenly a thought hit him. "Wait a minute—I didn't even realize it—do you know what tonight is?" he asked.

"Monday night?"

"No—yes—but it's the *yahrzeit*, the tenth anniversary of Rabbi Schneerson's death! I can't believe I forgot about this!"

Remember the rabbi who everyone thought might be the Messiah? Well, apparently he either wasn't, or else he was still working on it, because when he'd died ten years earlier, it sent the entire Lubavitch movement into a tailspin. It was a famous tradition on the anniversary night of his death to go to his grave, called The Ohel (the Hebrew name for a structure that lies over the burial place of a righteous person) at Montefiore Cemetery in Queens, and pray for the health of those you loved, believing that the Rebbe would hear and heed your prayers.

My parents had gone out there a few times, and asked me to join them, but I never did. I was down with Judaism, but that branch of Orthodoxy felt like it was almost a different religion than my own. I remained frustrated by the laws that separated men and women, both physically and culturally. I felt uncomfortable and guilty about my lack of traditional knowledge. Basically, it just wasn't my thing. I still felt guilty chanting in yoga class— "*Om shanti*"? Hi, Sanskrit. Not my religion! And my parents' God . . . not my God. I found it hypocritical to borrow their faith when I needed it, if I didn't plan to fully commit to it when times were good again. It was like asking the Tasti D-Lite counter guy to give you samples of three different flavors, but then you walk out the door without buying a cone. Or shopping for a pricy suit at Bloomingdale's, then wearing it with the tags on so that you can return it the next day (like I did when I dressed up as Monica). Except it's not some saleslady at Bloomic's you're pissing off, it's the LORD, and that ain't right! Or sleeping with a guy you don't really like when you know he cares about you. You never plan on seeing him again, but oh, it would be so good for tonight . . . He calls the next day, you blow him off. Maybe you can live with the guilt. Maybe you never see the guy again, and it's no big deal. But what if you're over it and he's not? What if he goes postal on you and the fury comes down? Except this is not just some *Fatal Attraction* thing, it's the wrath of GOD, and how do you expect that to feel? Not too good.

That's not how I roll. I don't borrow what I don't plan to return.

It's not that I don't respect religions that aren't my own. I appreciate the Catholics who ask Jesus to do me a solid, and the Wiccans who give offerings to Mother Earth on my behalf. So what if Jesus ain't my homeboy, or I don't vibe with the "magick" of the Goddess? Those sentiments have value to the person expressing them, and I find that incredibly moving. There are plenty of Lubavitchers who still pray for me every day, even those who don't know me personally (thank you, by the way). I could feel guilty about it, but they do it without expectation of reciprocation. In my personal way, I also pray for people who don't believe in prayer, not expecting anything from them in return. I'm a believer, but I prefer not to put a label on it. Nor do I insist on following an ancient set of rules to give my belief validity. If there is some all-powerful being at the controls, I'm asking God/BTP to borrow from my general karma account on their behalf. I believe there is an account. I don't feel like it's fair of me to take out a loan if I have no intention of ever paying it back, let alone investing money in the bank. You can't just mooch someone else's intense religious faith when you need it. True belief is having faith when you don't need it.

When Mick and I arrived at the kosher restaurant, it was Messiah Central: a Messiah carpool sign-up on the door, Messiah videotapes playing on the TV. The waiter was all, "Would you like a Messiah Burger?" It was like T.G.I. Friday's, except the buttons said: "TGIM: Thank God it's Messiah!" All these signs pointed toward Messiahville. All those people back in the Detroit shul were praying for me every day. Here I was telling my dad that

Celeste, the Third Eye Blind Lady, was trying to heal me, but I wasn't going to give his main man a chance?

Three hours later we'd checked MapQuest, rented a car, and were on our way to the cemetery. We left around midnight "to avoid the crowds," in Mick's words. It took us about forty minutes to drive to a modest neighborhood in Queens. We thought we were in the wrong place until suddenly . . . Mitzvah Mobiles were everywhere. Tour buses, Town Cars, cops, lighting rigs, news vans . . . and Lubies, Lubies, as far as the eye could see. Black hats, black coats, women in long sleeves and denim skirts, babies, everyone talking and yakking and gathering and greeting as if it were one in the afternoon and not one in the morning. Black and Hispanic neighbors were sitting out on their porches watching all this and going, "Damn!"

Mick and I pushed past suitcases and strollers, me trying not to make any body contact with anyone because, you know, I'm a woman and therefore impure at least once a month. We crossed through this tiny little house into a giant tent that was jam-packed with Jews. I glanced at my dad—he could have been at Yankee Stadium during the World Series for all the joy I saw in his eyes. The din was awesome—reunions, questions, directions, evaluations.

The tent was divided so the men were on one side milling around, and the women were packed into tables across the divider, writing their prayers in Hebrew on cream sheets of paper. Mick thrust some blank pages into my hand and said, "I'm gonna go find Rabbi Baumbacher. You stay here and write down your prayers. I'll be right back!" Off he went, a kid in a kosher candy store.

I sat across from three little girls, obviously sisters, one of whom stopped writing to ask the others, "Is it 'We want Messiah now' or did He already show up?" It's really easy to tell which daughters belong to which mothers. The gene pool is pretty small. Lubavitch kids are like those little Russian nesting dolls that you unpack: They all the look the same but each is just a bit smaller than the next, and there's always a tiny baby at the end. The teenage girls looked less like observant Jews than they did semi-cool counselors at Camp Seagull. "Hey, Rivke, what time is tie-dye today? . . . Great! See you at flag raising!"

Some of the younger moms were almost hip, yapping on Motorola cell phones they pulled from their fake Prada—or as I call it, Frauda—bags. They're not Orthodoxes, they're Orthofoxes! So I could tell there was still a social hierarchy in place. But as Myrn later explained to me, "Every single one of them ends up with a husband. Can you imagine how different your ego would be if you knew that no matter what you looked like, no matter how you dressed, you'd still end up a with a partner for life?" That must alleviate some self-esteem issues.

I sat down with my paper and my gel ink pen and started to write. I was ideally to do it in Hebrew of course, and say who I was and who my parents were. I knew that much: I'm Gitel Minya bat Sorah Esther (my Hebrew name, "daughter of" my mother's; when she got all Kabbalistic, Madonna chose Esther as her Jewish name). When I prayed for other people, I didn't know their Hebrew names or their parents' names . . . and half of 'em weren't even Jewish. I figured that I'd just have to wing it and let the Messiah sort it out later. Some women were filling reams and reams, but I didn't want to be greedy: God didn't have all night, so about a page and a half did it for me. I signed off, and then realized that I should really thank the rabbis for being so nice to my family. Recognize, ya know? So at the bottom I scrawled, "P.S. Big up to Rabbi Baumbacher and his family; they're doing a great job." I felt like I was filling out a customer service survey at Big Boy. I didn't know if the Rebbe knew what "big up" meant, but we were in Queens, after all.

My father was MIA. Some Orthofoxes in the corner were scolding a grandma whose grandbaby was howling. One literally yelled, Ratso Rizzo style, "Ay, we're trying to pray here!" Tough crowd, tough crowd. Hundreds milled around, thousands more outside, masses of people returning from the grave site with tears in their eyes. Mick was nowhere to be found. Tension was mounting. It was almost two in the morning. Suddenly I heard, "Wendy?"

It was Miriam and Shira Baumbacher, children nos. 3 and 2 in the Baumbacher clan! I hadn't seen them for years, but they recognized me. They'd just driven in from Michigan (a ten-hour ride) and came directly to the cemetery. "It's so great that you're here tonight," said sweet Shira, nineteen and already married almost a year. "The Rebbe always hears our prayers, but tonight it's like he's standing in front of God, reading them directly to him."

The girls pulled me through the crowd. I saw their dad waving us over from the divider in the tent. If I'd thought Mick was excited to be there, he had nothing on Rabbi Baumbacher. The man looked like he was at Jewish Disney World on his way to meet "Moishe" Mouse. Totally elated. "Eh, come this way," he said in his anachronistic Yiddish accent. "It's time now."

I got a quick glimpse of the man-only mob on his side of the tent before I stepped out the back door and found Mick. Somehow we got on the big *macher* VIP line. Good thing, too. Because even though it was the middle of the night, the way the cemetery was lit up I could see thousands of people shuffling step by step in line toward the tomb that housed the Rebbe's grave site. Men and women were separated by metal barricades, all gazing up at monitors where videotapes of the Rebbe speechifying played. It was eerily quiet out there after the din inside, hearing the dead man of honor speak. The only thing that broke up his words was the occasional shout through the megaphones by Israeli security guards. They yelled, "Keep moving, keep moving!" and "One way in and out!" and "Only two minutes inside the grave!" My dad and I wove among the gravestones and took our places opposite the huge line of people. I felt a momentary pang of Jewish guilt for taking cuts.

About forty people (of one gender at a time) could crush into the grave room, which was basically four cement walls with an open roof around the graves of the Rebbe and his father-in-law, who had been the previous leader of the movement. It was the men's turn, so there was a huge pile of black sneakers on the sidewalk. Kind of like yoga class at Kripalu or the Ayurvedic Institute. Mick pushed me forward as the men moved out and a group of women and children surged ahead. It did feel like Disney World—like when I was seven and my parents cajoled me into the arms of a giant Donald Duck, leaving me with a lifelong aversion to people dressed up in animal suits. Here, panicked, I shoelessly stepped down on a tiny path into the cement room, surrounded by women in wigs and tired little girls.

Inside the heavy walls were the two headstones, maybe eight feet tall and covered in Hebrew script. The stones themselves were surrounded by another cement wall, hip high, creating a pit. In the pit was paper. Tons and tons of ripped-up paper. Shredded prayers. A stunning visual representation of thousands of lives, thousands of wishes, the sick and the dying, the hopeful and the healing. No begging for Game Boys, no asking to lose weight. No digs at the president, no curiosity about Brangelina, no wishing for a new season of *Dancing with the Stars* to start already. Just pure, honorable prayer. Pop culture held no value here. Sincerity was what counted.

The women muttered under their breath, reading their letters out loud, then tore them up and threw them into the pit. I finished way before everyone else and looked around. Some were quietly rocking; some were openly weeping. One woman looked like she was so deep in the holy throes that she was going to pass out. It was hard for me to connect to the spirituality in the stress of it all—especially with the bellows of "Two minutes!" coming from the megaphones outside. They pushed us out to make room for the next group of men, so I ripped and tossed, smooshed outside, grabbed my New Balance kicks and headed back to the tent to find Mick.

Instead I found Rabbi Baumbacher chilling with Avram, Chaim, and Feivel (nos. 1, 6, and 4. Did I mention they had two sets of twins? Someone needs to give them a reality show). The rabbi still had his glow on, and began to share with me the significance of the tenth year after the Rebbe's death and why tonight was the biggest night and so on and so on . . . when I realized that I was hanging out on the men's side of the tent. "Is it okay for me to be on this side?" I asked him.

"Tonight," he responded with a gleam in his eye, "anything can happen."

Mick and I got back to my place at four in the morning. I couldn't sleep. Had that really gone down? Could it really make a difference? Would the Rebbe actually hear my prayers, and could he possibly respond, especially if I didn't follow the tenets of his religion? Turner, Rai, Lipman, and Prama had plenty to offer, but none of them had truly healed me. What if my true guru was Jewish? Maybe what I had always seen as the limitations of religion—the rules, the rituals, and the conservative thinking on gender—was somehow liberating. What a luxury it was to simply believe. Like having faith on autopilot. Autofaith.

A few days later I got some very good news from Turner. Seemed the last round of Rituxan treatment had been very effective. My blood tests came back A-OK. I didn't have to return and see him for another six weeks. It was welcome news.

Why did I get a pass that day? Certainly it could have been the medicine that did it. I liked to think the acupuncture was helping me too. Possibly Celeste had actually loosened up that blockage in my third eye. But what if it had been my little prayer at the Ohel that night, or the sum of the prayers that were being said for me every day in Lubavitch shuls, Catholic churches, and Muslim mosques across the country? Maybe there truly was a reason for everything; a reason why I was sick and a reason why I'd been born in the first place. Maybe the ability to heal myself was out of my control—and in the power of something greater. In that case I needed more than medicine; I needed to find the courage to believe.

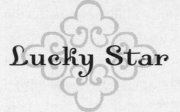

# Lucky Star

DECEMBER 6, 1983

MY 11TH BIRTHDAY (FLASHBACK EDITION)

CURRENT MUSIC:
MTV *is all* Thriller, *all the time (not that I know—Mick
won't let me and Josh watch MTV because he's
afraid we'll turn into "punk rockers")*

CURRENT LOOK:
*Fiorucci sweatshirt, neck cut off due to ongoing*
Flashdance *mania, acid green parachute
pants, pink patent leather shoes*

IN REGULAR NEWS:
*A guy named Bill Gates unveiled some
fancy computer software*

IN MADONNA NEWS:
*"Holiday," the third single from Madonna,
tops the charts*

At my eleventh birthday party, a psychic read my palm and revealed that someday . . . I'd collect thimbles. Very illuminating. I'm not sure why an honest-to-

God psychic was working kiddie birthday parties in West Bloom-field, Michigan, but I loved the idea that a person could be tapped into the future, witness to all the mysterious things that I couldn't see but hoped existed. I was fascinated by fairy tales and mystical objects like crystal balls and magic wands (but too superstitious to play around with Ouija boards). My interest in reincarnation came from the same zone.

When I was in my early twenties and working on an astrology television show at Lifetime, I had my first consultation with a real astrologer, Susan Miller. She explained what planets I had on my chart and what they meant (for those keeping track: I'm a Sagit-tarius, Aries rising, Leo moon). She told me, "You probably won't get married until your late thirties, but you've already met the man you are going to marry, back when you were about sixteen. He might be someone you work with, and he might have some sort of physical disability." I figure if a guy from my sophomore class at Andover High School in Bloomfield Hills rolls into my cubicle in a wheelchair, I'll pretty much have it made.

Astrology kicked off in the Babylonian era. Since sun, light, and rain came from the heavens and determined whether cul-tures would live or die, Babylonians assumed that the stars also clearly affected our lives. With no shortage of time on their hands, they divided the celestial sky into twelve sections, what we call the zodiac. Each section is associated with one month, one con-stellation, one animal, and one part of the human body (for example, Aries, the first sign, is the head; Pisces, the last sign, is the feet). Greeks, Romans, Hebrews, Persians, and Arabs supplemented the zodiac, while Chinese and Indians developed their own methodologies (Jyotish, for example, was the system Rai used). Through the Middle Ages and the Renaissance, astrology was considered a science. If Romeo and Juliet had simply had their charts done, they probably could have avoided a lot of trouble. Scientific advances led to the split between astronomy, the study of the stars and planets, and astrology, the skill of interpreting the present and predicting the future.

Astrology fascinated me in the same way mythology did. Cool stories, loved reading 'em, wish I remembered them better, helpful when doing literary analysis. But really, how could the date and time I was born truly affect my life? How could I share specific personality traits with other people just because I was born in December? Sure, elements of the Sagittarian profile seemed to suit me (eternal students, big talkers, searchers for the meaning of life), but others didn't (world travelers who love sports? nope). When I got that job writing on the astrology show, I really had to learn my Cancer from my Capricorn. The more I studied, the more astrology seemed to follow patterns. Mick was certainly a roaring Lion, while Myrn was such a balanced Libra. I found that I was drawn to Cancers, Leos, and Scorpios. I noticed that Cancers were attracted to parenting, while Scorpios generally were not (oh, but they were sexy MF's, those Scorps). My sun (Sagittarius), moon (Leo), and rising sign (Aries) were all fire signs, which matched up with my Jyotish chart. I often butted heads with people of other fire signs, or felt doused out by water signs. I began to view astrology as emotional meteorology: Years of study show that when the sun is here, and the temperature is this, and it's this time of year, it's going to rain. It's up to you whether you want to bring an umbrella.

The trick for me was deciphering the reliable horoscopes from the capricious (unpredictable, like a Capricorn!). For every job offer that was accurately foretold to me by some mystic, the romance-to-be never came through. Maybe I'd go on the trip they predicted, but I wouldn't win a projected cash windfall. Still, for all my grains of saltiness, I couldn't help but keep an eye on the calendar on days when my horoscope forecasted a bountiful job offer, or a soulmate expected at the door. Especially if he was in a wheelchair.

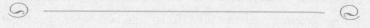

OCTOBER 2005

Since I was in a period of health equilibrium, I yearned for some input about what to do with my life aside from enduring Wegener's. My friend Lynn hooked me up with Jenny Lynch, the astrologer from *Glamour* magazine. I'd read her material for years, and thought Jenny had a very balanced sensibility about this inconsistent art form.

She'd studied with the best in the business for years, but Jenny says that her interest in astrology started when she was a little girl. As a Leo, she was fascinated with lions. She started paying attention to all things feline. As she went through childhood travails, she found comfort in scrutinizing the stars. In the 1970s she studied with some famous astrologers and realized within her first few professional readings that she had a knack for this stuff. As she examines a chart, Jenny says she gets different feelings and images that she expresses to the client. Whether it's about money, relationships, or where one should live, her predictions are savvy and sometimes eerily accurate. Most of all, she's a really good listener. Between the information she can gather from a chart, and talking to the client one-on-one, she gives excellent advice.

I went to Jenny's apartment on St. Marks Place in the East Village for a reading (just a block south of the Wicca witch shop, I noted). These were the streets Madonna had strolled when she first moved to New York, and when she was shooting *Desperately Seeking Susan*. I even passed Love Saves the Day, the store where Madonna trades Susan's pyramid jacket for those studded boots, on the way over to Jenny's place. Jenny was blond, with a fit yoga body that made her look twenty years younger than her actual age. The front room was painted red and filled with drums, books, and tarot cards. Two big computer monitors were set up in the back bedroom, where I sat down as if I were about to do a TV edit. Jenny confirmed my birth info and popped my chart up on her screen. It looked like a big ring divided into twelve sections, with little symbols dotted around the ring that I recognized as planets. "Your sun up here is in the sign of Sagittarius, with Jupiter, which is the sign of a pretty much optimistic person." She tapped the top of the chart. "The sun also represents the father. You should have had a nice father. Did you?"

"Yes," I said. "He's great." Sometimes Lubavitchery, but great.

"Is he a teacher?" she asked.

He taught me how to ride a bike, but I didn't think that was what Jenny meant. "No, he was a gourmet food distributor in Michigan. But he's been retired for a while."

"Really? Because according to this chart, he may be a guru."

"My *dad?*"

"Yes, wait and see."

Wow. Maybe I'd been searching for all the answers everywhere but the first place I needed to go. Mickey Shanker, mezuzah-loving guru. Jenny continued: "Because your sun sign is Jupiter, you're very lucky. Oh, imagine if I had that in my horoscope every day. . . . I only get it once a year. I thought you would be a writer because you have the sun in Jupiter and Mercury in the ninth house of publishing, and Saturn, the planet of destiny, is in the sign of Gemini. It's a signature for a career in communication."

Jenny paused. "There's something really strange going on with your horoscope." Strange, strange, I liked strange. I yearned to be told that I was actually an Egyptian princess, or the owner of a golden tiara and a mysterious invisible plane.

"Saturn is opposed to Neptune, and you have so many planets up in the ninth house of the higher mind. That means you're searching for a spiritual understanding of life, but Neptune, the planet of dreams and illusion, doesn't make it easy. I think you're going to go through a huge transformation in the next two years. Eventually you're going to become a spiritual teacher. But that's a few years away. There's a definite search to integrate spirituality into your work, because of this Saturn/Neptune opposition."

"I'm going to be a spiritual teacher?" Unless I was going to teach people how to be spiritually ambivalent and/or cynical, that path seemed unlikely. But the "few years away" idea was appealing; maybe that meant I would make it past thirty-five. I hadn't mentioned my health problems to Jenny. I was curious to see if they'd show up on my chart.

Jenny resumed. "You don't really have many emotional problems showing up in your horoscope. It's a very clean slate. You have a couple of challenges, but not many planets confronting each other, so your karma's pretty clean. Mercury, the planet of communication, rules the way you think and you're very much a high-minded person. Mercury is in Sadge and it's retrograde and it's very strong. In the ninth house of publishing." She pointed to a copy of *The Fat Girl's Guide* that I had brought her as a gift. "This is a great start, this book here, but I think you're going to write more serious books."

In a way, Jenny was doing the same thing a doctor did: reading a chart, interpreting it, and giving me a prognosis. What a pleasure to have an expert tell me who I was and what I was going to do so I didn't have to figure it out all by myself!

Jenny: "There's a wound showing up as Chiron in the first house. It means that you'll be a pioneer in the healing arts. Because it's in the sign of Aries, that means you yourself may have a wound." She sat back from the screen and turned to me. "Do you know much about Chiron?"

I had a dusty memory from trying to memorize Edith Hamilton's *Mythology* in the eleventh grade. I answered, "I know it's a faraway planet. And that mythologically, it's the story of a centaur who was wounded and abandoned by his parents, but he grew up to be a wise man and a healer."

Jenny nodded. "When it's on your ascendant, or the planet that was coming over the horizon at the moment you were born, that's your body or your self. So it means *you* have the wound. Once you heal the wound, then you can teach others the technique."

"A physical wound?" I asked.

"Often it is, but it can be emotional, too. Let me tell you about Chiron in the first house." She clicked on the symbol and read from her computer program. "'You are wounded either emotionally or physically and every time you express your essential being you experience rejection. This may lead to self-exploration and later on you may become a wounded healer or a teacher.' So one of the problems is that there's some kind of wound that needs to be healed. Emotional or physical, probably a little of both.

"There's also another wound coming up with the love life." Of course there was. "Chiron squared to Venus. Planets that are squared are like opposing forces." Jenny clicked her mouse again. How did astrologers do this analysis before computers? On a freakin' abacus? "Now it talks about a painful relationship: 'You experience emotional pain in your relationships, you have difficulty experiencing the joy and beauty of intimate relationships. You need to face early childhood feelings of rejection and develop empathy for those close to you.'" A shrink couldn't have said it any better. That's the great thing about astrology: It's like two years of therapy smushed into one hour. Jenny could not only tell me what was wrong with me, but also assure me it was all going to work out famously in the end. Et tu, Freud? I hoped her chart wouldn't reveal the same "curtailed life" length that Rai's had. Then again, he'd told me I needed to "forgive" in order to get well; that was awful close to "facing childhood feelings of rejection and developing empathy" for people I loved.

Jenny paused. "I want to ask you. . . . Have you had a head injury? As I mentioned, Chiron—that's the wounded healer—is in Aries, which rules the head."

A head injury? That was one way of putting it. I filled Jenny in on my health sitch. "Over the last couple of years, I got this rare autoimmune disease. It made me crazy ill. It started in my sinuses, then went to my lungs, then it eventually moved into my eyes and ears and nose and the lining of my brain. I'd say that counts as a head injury."

Jenny nodded and clicked again on the screen. "If we look at Chiron in Aries it says, 'Your sense of well-being has been violated. In a way, you feel afraid of asserting yourself. You'll also overcompensate by being the first at everything. Physically you may suffer head wounds. You may become a pioneer in a way which will be of service to humanity.' That's one of your main agenda things; it has to do with healing. It may not seem like an attractive thing to you at this age but you're still very young. You are going to be going through a big spiritual development for many reasons over the next year. Neptune is over here in your fifth house, and it's going to be sextiling your Jupiter."

I'd always wondered what it felt like to get my Jupiter sextiled.

Jenny's face lit up with excitement. "This is going to bring a lot of stimulation. It's almost like your mind opens up to receive a higher vibration of thought. . . . Something is going to happen. Something interesting. I don't know exactly what, but I would think that you will have ability, focus. It could be a study or a writing project, possibly a book. Your mind is going to be super-powerful when it comes to intellectual stuff, and writing. So the beginning is March 2006—and the transit lasts all the way until July 2007. Pluto on your Mercury. Pluto is the planet of intensity, depth, focus. You may decide to study something that's like a mystery. Could have something to do with past-life regression, or the occult. One of the good things about this is that it's an emotionally maturing time. And after you go through this you'll never be a baby again. You may cry a lot during this period, but after that it's going to be over."

Always good to know that excessive weeping has an end date.

Jenny picked up my book and looked at it again. "Did you do your book tour in the States? Because . . ." She pointed to a globe that appeared on the computer screen. "I saw some good lines here. This is called astral cartography.

"You have a karmic connection line going through the San Francisco area. If you go there you might meet people you feel you were destined to meet." Tracy lived outside San Francisco. Maybe there were other special people she'd introduce to me to, like her healers out there.

Jenny continued: "Your perfect holiday lines are in India."

"No!"

"You're not going there now, but someday, you might."

Hilarious. Maybe if I went to India I could meet Dr. Rai's best friend, the tree.

Jenny ran her finger over a different spot on the map. "If you go to this line here they say you'll get money. So let's see where that is. . . . That line would be in . . . "

"Albuquerque!" I interrupted.

"No, it's more like Phoenix, Sedona. . . ."

"I can't be one of those Sedona people." That was Gray Braid/ screen door central. We both laughed. Jenny continued. "This is what they say: If you are seeking a more spiritual or artistic direction this can be a good line to follow."

I paid Jenny a hundred and fifty dollars for her services; well worth it. She offered to stay in touch. She knew that I, being a Sadge, was into learning, so she suggested some books I could buy in the used bookstore down her street. I began to study astrology in earnest. Now I had a new path to pursue: Go through some pain (check), fix the wounds (working on it), and become a spiritual healer in Sedona (yikes). It was just what I'd always never dreamed of.

# 12

# Express Yourself

NOVEMBER 2005

y liver enzymes continued to fluctuate as I maintained my Wegener's halfsies treatment (half East, half West). I started to get stomachaches so bad that I doubled over in pain, and didn't want to eat. One morning I woke up and looked in the mirror and noticed that my eyes were yellow. Sticky-pad yellow. Second chakra yellow, which was the chakra related to digestive problems. Jaundice. However, my bowel movements had no color. They looked like Silly Putty. Apparently both my eyes and my excretions were being sponsored by the gummy department at 3M. I *basti*'d myself silly.

I noticed that my clothes were a little loose on me. At first I thought it was due to the steroid inflammation settling down, and the stomach upset I felt every time I ate. Then pounds started pouring off me. I lost almost forty pounds in a nine-week period.

For a woman who had built a career on fat positivity, my weight loss was torturous. Because most people in the world are complete twits, I was continually congratulated for losing weight, several doctors included. When I aired my concerns about the sudden loss to one expert, he clapped me on the shoulder and suggested, "Won't it be fun to go shopping for new jeans?" Oh yes, he did. If it had been a couple of pounds here or there, I get it. But forty pounds in two months? That constitutes a medical emergency.

All those years I'd wanted to lose weight; now I'd lost so much weight—the equivalent of an entire Nicole Richie—when I didn't want to. I was maybe one of the handful of women on the planet who accepted my (over)weight. It was an ongoing process, and it wasn't easy. But hell, I'd written a book about it and finally felt decent in my skin.

Now I became terrified of readers seeing me and saying, "But you're not fat." Oh, I was fat, I just wasn't fat *enough*. If there was one thing that irritated me about certain celebrity body acceptance icons, it was their hypocrisy. I couldn't take one more chubby starlet telling *Access Hollywood* that all was right in her world . . . and then watch her get liposuction live on TV. They had their fat sucked out, their breasts hacked off, they stopped eating, they took pills, they did gastric bypass surgery, they blamed their sudden change in appearance on age or dehydration or some other nonsense. It wasn't about the numbers; everyone is entitled to make her own choices about her body. It was about lying to themselves. Don't tell me you're proud of your curves and then have a Beverly Hills surgeon remove them.

When I was promoting the book, people would ask, "If you

could magically wake up thin tomorrow, wouldn't you want to?" It wasn't that the answer was an unequivocal no; the question was simply no longer relevant. I'd stopped imagining an alternate life of razor-sharp cheekbones and razor-thin stiletto heels. I no longer assumed that the reason I didn't get the things I wanted—the job, the money, the love—was my weight. So there's the twist: When I finally feel good about my weight, I lose it.

Intuitives and shrinks have a field day with this one. The metaphor is too rich to resist: I no longer needed the weight so I dumped it. I was opening up, peeling back defenses, discovering that the root of my problems wasn't a lack of immunity to cheesecake, but my immune system itself.

Maybe I would have felt satisfaction or comfort if I became a smaller version of myself as I lost weight. But I didn't. It was like someone had attached a hose to my well-proportioned body and sucked all the air out. I was like a sack of skin. I never understand why people on *The Biggest Loser* and in weight loss commercials who lose hundreds of pounds have perfect skin tautly stretched over their new, tawny muscles. No human skin is that elastic. I have so many stretch marks that it looks like a tiger clawed me. I guess their luck has something to do with scalpels or the magic of Photoshop.

Plus everything was in the wrong place. My hips slunk down to my thighs, my boobs went south, my armpits dangled somewhere on the middle of my torso. Nothing fit right. They don't make Spanx for that.

I had a closet full of glamorous outfits that no longer fit. I believed in spending money on designers who made elegant plus-size clothes, so a lot of my stuff was expensive. Right before I got sick I'd commissioned a craftastic artist to make me a hand-knit, full-length shawl. I picked out the colors: pink, turquoise, purple. It was expensive but it was going to be like my superhero cape. By the time she finished, it hung on me like a wet poncho. I was down to about 178 pounds.

Going shopping was not a pleasure. I was too small for plus sizes but too large for straight fits. Oh, the plight of the average woman, the size 14 who can't find a home in a department store. The homeless guy on my corner was appreciative of my new silhouette, however. He was an older African-American man, maybe a little slow, with eyes that looked in two different directions. He had a habit of wanting to kiss my hand after I gave him money, which was a very sweet gesture but also made me concerned about where that mouth had been. One day as I stood on the corner waiting for the light to change, he looked at me and said appraisingly, "You know, I'll eat a burger with or without the bun. But miss, you look mighty fine without the bun!"

I got plenty of compliments that made me feel awful. They weren't complimenting me; they were complimenting my illness. It was all so wrong.

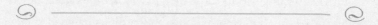

JANUARY 2006

I took another battery of blood tests: My liver enzyme levels were psychotic. It made no sense; Wegener's generally didn't affect the liver. My skin was the color of butterscotch pudding. I couldn't digest or expel. I had bruises everywhere, and tiny little spider veins crept all over my chest. My abdomen was unbearably tender to the touch. I was losing weight like the guy from that Stephen King book *Thinner*. But a gypsy had cursed that dude. Only two words could explain all those symptoms: liver cancer.

I had myself a nice little Google fest to get acquainted with the disease that I was sure was killing me. Liver cancer is one of the worst cancers, now that our society is so cancer-friendly that you can rank cancers from "Incredibly treatable!" (thyroid) to "Have you talked to anyone at Sloan-Kettering?" (pancreas).

The bell went off and my hunt began to find the Number One Hepatologist in the World. Fatty Liver Boy and Jason the Biopsy Serial Killer were out. Another snide physician told me vitamins were to blame. Finally, all roads pointed toward a doctor in New York who was world renowned and well respected, a liver specialist who could surely figure out how to make me well. Turner pulled strings and I ended up in his office right before Christmas (why do I always have a crisis at Christmas?). He was reserved and seemed thoughtful and self-assured. As he looked over my charts and listened to my description of the last few months, I could see him running through the differentials in his mind. I paused before saying, "I'm pretty sure. . . . I mean, it's gotta be liver cancer, right?"

Number One had a good hearty laugh over that one. "No way," he assured me. "This isn't cancer. I'm ninety-nine percent sure that you've got something called primary sclerosing cholangitis, which is a blockage in your bile ducts. Basically bile is not getting to your liver, so your liver can't do its job, which is filtering toxins and aiding digestion. We'll clear out the ducts and you'll be fine."

More duct cleaning, but from a different direction than the *basti*. I appreciated his explanation and admired his confidence. He ordered me to have a few exploratory scans and scopes before he could go in and clear those ducts—MRCP, ERCP, endoscopy, colonoscopy, biopsy, etc.—but he estimated that by the end of January everything was going to be in working order again. I felt relieved to hand over the reins of diagnosis and decision making to the Best Guy. Maybe he was the one who would finally make me better.

The scope results showed his diagnosis was incorrect: It wasn't primary sclerosing cholangitis, or a similar disease called primary biliary cirrhosis. Luckily he hadn't found any malignancies. There was a tubular adenoma in my colon, but we could definitively rule out liver cancer. As we disproved theory after theory, I had the distinct feeling that Number One was frustrated with me for ruining his diagnostic hepatology batting average. He finally threw up his hands and gave me a diagnosis of autoimmune hepatitis. Autoimmune. Again my body was screwing up my body. My system hadn't delivered what he predicted, which was a blockage of some kind. No chance he could be wrong. Instead he placed the fault squarely on me and my irascible liver.

As it turns out, my liver is named Laverne.

While traveling on my not-always-healing journey, I

went to lots of seminars and guided meditations where I was told
to look inside my body and see myself, visually identify discomfort
or pain, or make a connection between the internal and external.
Another kind of meditation. That never worked for me. First
of all, I don't like closing my eyes in front of rooms full of strang-
ers. Even when I did, the most I ever saw was red, just the color
red, because if you cut me open a whole lot of red would come
out. Also, when you close your eyes and see light through your
eyelids, you are essentially looking at blood-tinged skin. Clearly,
imagery was not my strong suit. I could never draw. I liked letters
and words, not pictures. When healers told me to imagine I was
walking along a beach, the best I could drum up was an image of
seabirds drowned in the *Exxon Valdez* oil spill who had washed up
on the sand; I didn't think that's what they had in mind. I'm a
terrible, easily distracted meditator, but to this day I keep trying.

While being scoped and prodded by the liver doc, I went to
see a craniosacral practitioner named Alora. An osteopathic mo-
dality invented in the twentieth century, craniosacral therapists
use their hands to manipulate tissues around the brain, spinal
cord, and central nervous system to get the body working more
efficiently. It was also supposed to help ease the negative effects
of emotional turmoil. At that point I was drained. I felt toxic, the
docs were driving me mad, and I was willing to try any therapy
that didn't involve talking or paperwork.

Alora had a warm, trustworthy demeanor, kind eyes, blond
hair, and a beautiful smile. She radiated positive energy, making
me feel like I was in safe hands. Alora had led twelve different
lives (literally and figuratively, as she was certain we'd met in a

previous life)—as a production manager on movies, a marketing executive, a cricket farmer—but injuries from a car accident led her to body work. In her free time she was studying with a Chinese Zen master who was teaching her to walk through walls. While I lay on a massage table, she gently cradled the back of my head in her hands and assessed a lot of trouble in the liver. "Have you ever tried to talk to your liver?" she asked. I wasn't aware that as CEO of my body, I had to contact my liver in the first place. "Nah," I said, "but be my guest if you guys want to chat."

"Just consider it," she urged me. "Try to open up some communication with your body." I didn't want communication. My patience had run out. I wanted a problem fixed, and that's what I was paying Alora $180 (not covered by insurance) to do. As she lightly manipulated my body, I'd rest on her table and look outside the window onto a secret garden in the middle of Manhattan. Even with my crappy hearing, I could hear birds chirping. Occasionally three little birds would alight on a tree branch and watch Alora treat me. My refusal to dialogue with my digestive tract would be our opener when I would stop by for a session each week. "Have you talked to your liver yet?" Alora would ask. "Nope, not yet," I'd respond, swinging my legs up. "It's all yours."

On the M.D. side, there was nothing but bad news: awful blood tests getting awfuler; a digestive system that had crashed and burned. I was still losing weight. Number One, the liver expert, was directing me to take higher doses of steroids. But in Alora's room, things were a bit better. We became very comfortable with each other. I started to refer to my liver as "Laverne," as in, "No, I still haven't had a conversation with Laverne. Sorry, Alora."

When I finally caved and began to kibitz with my internal organs, I did it as a joke. "Okey dokey smokey, I'm a-gonna talk to my liver now, ha ha ha." I thought it would make for an entertaining story to tell my friends. Technically a liver looks like a bloody slab of whatever the biggest meat is in the butcher's case at the local Safeway, but I gave that slab a personality. I pictured Laverne as an older black woman, maybe in her early sixties, short on chitchat and big on efficiency. In my imagination, she often added colorful scarves or decorative brooches to accent her conservative suit from Talbot's. She wore a wig and no one had ever seen her without it. She went to church and belonged to several church committees including "Tyler Perry Movie Night" and "Jesus Loves a Book Club." In my mind, Laverne had two adult kids (son married, daughter divorced) and three grandchildren who lived in Texas and Florida. She was hoping to retire soon and maybe move down near, say, St. Augustine herself.

I envisioned her minding her own, managing my body's filtering business as she always had, when suddenly it went off the rails. Sure, she'd had to do some overtime in the last couple of years when those chemicals (steroids, chemo, antibiotics) had been dumped in my system. As if she didn't have enough to manage, what with that flamboyant nitwit Steve the Spleen goofing off all the time, and only the most minimal communication with Gail, my gall bladder. ("What is wrong with Gail?" I imagined some of the other organs whispering to each other in the break room. "What is her blockage? She needs to go outside and get a little color in her cheeks, a little vitamin D in her system. No one is ever going to want to hang out with a gall bladder with that sallow complexion.")

The more detail I gave to my organs, the harder it was to pretend they were just body parts. I recognized that Laverne's well-planned, well-executed systems, which had been working efficiently in my body for more than thirty years, had screeched to a halt. Some God-knows-what hooligan cells created by my immune system showed up and made a shambles out of Laverne's entire workplace. At first she probably thought it was some sort of practical joke from Thelma the Thyroid or one of her glandular friends, poking holes in her walls or scrambling up her enzymes. It wasn't Thelma. It was me—my grief/lack of forgiveness/lack of effort/ overmedication/extremism/imbalance, depending on which guru I spoke to. To think, Laverne had been that close to retirement. . . .

It wasn't a joke anymore. I owed my body an apology. While I recharged on Alora's table, I silently offered a message to my liver: "Sorry, Laverne."

It was a begrudging breakthrough. Alora explained that Laverne felt put out because all I did was rag on her when she'd been working so hard all this time. So each week I'd say, "Laverne, I owe you some TLC. I'm grateful for all you've done so far. But bad news—here we go again." For lack of a better consensus, Number One was sticking with that diagnosis of autoimmune hepatitis. The treatment plan was a major steroid boost, plus Imuran. The verdict still didn't add up to me: If steroids would make me better, and I'd been increasing steroids, shouldn't my liver be improving? Plus the weight loss hadn't stopped. I'd lost sixty-two pounds in a matter of months. If I ever doubted my assertion that weight loss was not the definition of happiness, I knew for sure now. It sucked. The pants hanging off my flattened ass were definitive proof that I'd rather be fat and healthy than not-so-fat and sick. Still, one acquaintance eyed me admiringly. "I didn't *want* to lose the weight," I blustered. "It's because my liver isn't working. I'm *ill*."

"Still," she said under her breath. "Isn't it worth it?"

No, lady. It ain't.

Once I broke the dam by dialoguing with Laverne, it was easy to give all of my organs their own personalities. I once watched an entire *Oprah* about vaginal self-esteem ("Who has it and how to get it"). But what about pancreatic faith? Hematological confidence? Maybe we were spending too much time and energy working on our relationships with our vulvas when it was our lungs that really needed our love.

The bad symptoms began to ease up. The liver enzyme numbers improved. And my visits with Alora and the chitchat with my body parts led me to the next step I had to take.

I'd deferred to authorities in so many arenas, hoping they could fix me. Traditional Western medicine with Turner. A whole different form of traditional medicine with Rai. Prama's sensible suggestions, Jenny's visionary abilities, even Alora's guidance. Then Number One's history of hepatological success stories. There had to be someone who knew the answers and could give me the quick fix. They were experts in their respective fields.

But I was the expert on me. When I finally listened, my body gave me the answers. Laverne & Company spelled it out: "Wendy, stop taking the medication." I'd been warned many times not to quit steroids cold turkey. That could lead to adrenal shock (Arthur the Adrenal Gland was an old Yid). The synthetic cortisol provided by prednisone had replaced my natural adrenal function. It would take months for the adrenals to learn to work on their own again; in the meantime I would have completely unregulated cortisol and adrenaline function. That could send my body into a free fall that would end badly. Plus I was afraid that the Wegener's would rage without any medication.

Even so. With Alora nodding and the three little birds chirping approvingly in the background, I finally considered ignoring medical direction completely and tapering off the meds. It was Laverne and me in cahoots. Our mind-body partnership was brilliant. We deserved a bonus.

# 13

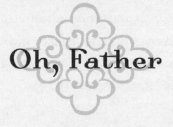

# Oh, Father

FEBRUARY 2006

I went to Alora religiously for craniosacral treatments, popped my vitamins, got poked by acupuncture needles, and felt better than I had in a long, long time. I was still on plenty of prednisone but had begun the gradual process of tapering off.

Mick and Myrn were less than thrilled with my decision to dismiss the doctors' game plan, and explore complementary and alternative paths. I was very confident with my choices about conventional medicine and unconventional measures. But I understand how hard it must be for the circle of people one step removed from the chronically ill patient to be supportive. They're either too involved or not involved enough. They ask you for information and then blanch when you share the gory details. They cheer you on your course of action, then question why you haven't tried something else. Every family is different, and every

243

patient has a different strategy. If I have any advice to the circle it's this: Do your best to wait to be asked for help or advice. If you really see your parent or child or partner make a life-risking choice, you have every right to jump in there. But if not, trust that the patient is the authority, bite your tongue, cross your fingers, and when in doubt, supply baked goods.

I flew down to visit my parents in Miami. Mick picked me up outside baggage claim. The second I got in the car, he dropped a bomb on me. We hadn't even pulled away from the curb when he started speaking excitedly. "I have an idea. I don't think you're going to like it. It's an ancient Jewish cure, and it's been done for thousands of years." (Later, I Googled this. If such a thing exists, there was no record of it on Google.) He continued: "You take a pigeon and you put it on you, and the pigeon takes away all the disease, and you just keep putting pigeons on you until the disease is gone, and that's it."

Maybe I'd misunderstood. "Put pigeons on me?"

"Yeah, you put the pigeons on you and they take away the disease."

"Why pigeons? Why not woodpeckers? Or bluebirds?" (Chicken, Jewish. Pigeon, not Jewish. Duck, Jewish. Swan, not Jewish.)

"I don't know."

I tried another tactic. "How do the pigeons take away the disease?"

"They suck it out of you."

"With their beaks? Like through my belly button?"

"No, you put the pigeons *on* you."

As if I should have a visual of what that looks like. I was now guessing he wanted me to place a pigeon on my torso. My inner vegetarian had a question. "What happens to the pigeons?"

"Oh . . . they take on the disease and they die."

"They die?"

He waved the question away. "I assume they die."

I pictured an African witch doctor grabbing a squawking chicken who knows it's about to have its throat cut, wings flapping in the air and feathers flying, dust kicking up, drums beating, Lisa Bonet hopping around, straight out of *Angel Heart.* "How many pigeons does it take?"

Now my dad was getting frustrated with me. "As many as it takes. The rabbi can give you all these details."

"Where am I supposed to get them? Central Park?"

"I don't know about the pigeons, all these details with the pigeons. The rabbi will call you. All I know is that it's an ancient Jewish cure, and it works."

I envisioned bearded rabbis bending over me as I lay in my dining room, the table covered in a white sheet, pigeon carcasses dropping and littering the parquet floor. I asked, "Have you spoken to anyone who has put pigeons on themselves?"

"No."

"Then how do you know it works?"

He spoke like *I* was the one who'd lost it. "Because it *does.*"

I'd dripped oil on my forehead, stuck needles in my skin, chatted with my gastrointestinal tract, shined colored lights on my chakras, and seriously considered drinking Emmy and Carrie's breast milk. (In a nonpasteurized form, human breast milk is supposed to be a natural immune booster. But I thought that their babies needed it more than I did, and that if for some reason I died, my friends would never forgive themselves.) In the hierarchy of nonsensical things that I'd tried in the name of health, there was no reason pigeon putting was worse than anything else. But the "pigeons + ancient Jewish cure + lack of proof" combo was simply too much for me to accept. I had limits. Intentional animal sacrifice was one of them. I certainly wasn't going to rub nasty, dirty pigeons all over me and watch them die. What would I do with them? Dump them in the garbage and expect the sanitation department to pick them up at the curb? Besides, I still felt guilty about taking any tips from my father's spiritual advisers. It was like the Ohel situation again. I refused to be a believer when I was in trouble but a skeptic when I wasn't in the mood.

"I'm sorry, Dad, but there is no way I am putting pigeons on me."

He pleaded, "You haven't even talked to the rabbi yet. You don't know."

"This crosses a line. This is voodoo. I'm not going to kill birds to fix my liver, and that's that."

Clearly Mick was displeased. Here he'd found a perfect solution for my problem and I wouldn't even consider it. We parked the car with the valet at their Miami apartment building. Myrn opened the apartment door with an expectant look. "Did Daddy tell you about the pigeons?"

"Yes, he did. I'm not doing it. I'm sorry, that's the end of the discussion."

"Fine, fine," she said with a shrug. It was an ancient Jewish shrug born in shtetls across Eastern Europe and featured frequently in *Fiddler on the Roof*. "It's your body," she sighed. "You know best." But for the entire trip, every time a pigeon would alight (which they did surprisingly often in Miami), my parents looked at me as if to say, "See? It's a sign."

M y parents drove me back to the airport on Friday afternoon, in time for them to go home and prepare for Shabbat. I left them with a warning: "I do not want any rabbis calling me. You understand? Do not give out my number." They muttered promises and I flew home. Like a pigeon.

I returned from the heat of Miami to a frozen slab of New York City. On the cab ride home from LaGuardia, the taxi driver blared Bob Marley: *"Don't worry about a thing….Every little thing's gonna be all right…."*

I couldn't help but worry. My life was worry. My focus had to be on illness, and I resented it. I longed for a normal life of carefree beer drinking and boundless energy that all the other people my age seemed to have. Every decision I made had to be filtered through Wegener's, whether it was what food to eat, or what vitamins to take, or whom to hang out with. Flying on a plane was practically a DEFCON 3 situation. But finally, I was home. So relieved to be in my apartment. I hit the playback button on my answering machine.

*Wendy, it's Rabbi Schwartz in Miami. You father gave me your number upon my request.*

The rabbi had that same lilting, Jewish, Brooklyn-inflected vocal pattern that I'd heard from other Lubavitchers. I thought I'd made it clear to my parents that no dirty bird application shall be done unto me. But here was the rabbi, calling with specific pigeon-purchase bullet points:

*Call a pet shop in Manhattan. Give them a credit card, ask them what they charge for per bird, ask them to tape it for you, pay them extra for that. Those birds are clean, but they can clean it up better with warm soap and water. They can disinfect it. All they do is tape up the legs with simple white tape, the legs and the feet with white tape, so they shouldn't flap around. And in one minute the whole thing can be resolved. It's a matter of superabsorbance that only pigeons have, to liver ailments on body contact, not in reverse. Ask them to send them in a taxi, or have someone to bring them over, it should be an eighteen-, twenty-, thirty-dollar delivery charge, and that's that.*

Let me get this straight: This mystery pet shop owner was supposed to messenger over a cage of pigeons in the back of a taxicab? Plus no one was even going to come by and help me with this procedure? I was supposed to put on pigeons by myself?

> *Try to get it done before Shabbos. It's a special week, especially for miraculous kinds of health cures. The Torah speaks specifically about this week more than any other time. The most important thing is, I insist you should be well. I pray that HaShem should give you a blessing as well, and I called the Rebbe today, and everything should turn out, you should definitely make sure to make every effort that there should be improvement. Everything good for you. Bye.*

I was confused. He said he'd called the Rebbe, the same one whose grave I visited with my father, the one who died in 1994. Maybe it was a figure of speech, as in, he called upon the Rebbe . . . in prayer. Who knows, maybe he literally phoned him. There could be some sort of Lubavitcher Rebbe hotline that outsiders didn't have access to without a special code from AT&T.\*

I did not call the pet store and pay a premium to get taped-up pigeons. I went out with my friends and saw *Brokeback Mountain* instead. When I returned home late on Saturday night, the machine was blinking.

---

\* As it turns out, there is. The rabbis have a direct dial to a guy at the Ohel. He writes down the appeal and a rabbinical student runs it over to the grave site, where he says a prayer, tears up the paper and puts it in the Rebbe's grave, as I had done.

*Wendy, a gute vach.* It's Rabbi Schwartz. I'm just curious*
*if you got the pigeons before the snow started. I read up more*
*about this custom a whole Shabbos. It seems to be very accurate*
*for anyone who has any kind of jaundice, not necessarily any*
*other problem, any kind of yellowish appearances in the eyes or*
*the face, and it seems to be very clear. Be well; let's hear good*
*news. Bye.*

On Sunday I called the rabbi back and left a polite message, saying that while I no longer planned to follow doctor's orders, I already had my own alternatives in mind. Thanks but no thanks. I thought the discussion was over—until Friday afternoon rolled around the following week. I saw Miami area code 305 pop up on the caller ID and I let the machine take it.

*Wendy, hi, good afternoon, it's Rabbi Schwartz, your*
*father's friend.*

Sigh. How did I go from having everything all figured out to being alone in my apartment listening to a rabbi berate me about pigeons on my answering machine?

*God should honor you with a perfect refueh shlaima.†*
*That's more important—that's equally important to the*

---

* "Have a good week," a traditional post-Shabbat greeting.
† Healing prayer.

*medicine. There's a spiritual aspect of every organ, there's a spiritual aspect to life. It's spiritual; you can't inherently hold it. Emotions are spiritual; our soul is certainly empirical. It's real, it's tangible, it's everlasting, and you're everlasting and good and wonderful; good things that you do are always going to be with you.*

Something stirred in me. Maybe this guy was on to something. Rai, Lipman the acupuncturist, Prama, Alora . . . they would all sign on with the spiritual organ theory. I could tell the rabbi spoke from his heart.

*I'm sorry; I'm not trying to interfere. I'm only trying to help. Because your dad is a sweet, delightful, wonderful person and I'm sure you are, too. I wish you an enormous amount of well-being, health and happiness, and everything else you can imagine that's excellent for you. You should feel spiritually comfortably and physically comfortably and everything comfortably. Thank you.*

I sat down on my living room floor and cried.

I got it. It didn't matter if what he suggested made sense. It didn't even matter if it worked. He believed it did, and that was enough. All of the people I'd met felt the same way. They were generous enough to open up their beliefs and practices to me, even if I resisted. The same for my parents. They didn't need proof. They had faith. Nothing was going to work if I didn't believe in it. I always thought I was like Wendy in *Peter Pan*. Turns out I was

Tinkerbell. If I wanted to believe in myself, I had to start clapping out loud.

On a later trip to Florida (after berating my parents for giving out my phone number), I met Rabbi Schwartz. He was, as I'd imagined, full of warmth and good intentions. A believer. He never tried to make me feel bad about skipping Operation Pigeon. He was just happy that my health had improved. But every time I get a bad test result, or a stomachache, and the tremor of "Oh, no, what if . . ." runs through me, I have to think: What if they were right? What if the solution to all this health drama was to grab a pigeon and rub it around on me, and in a minute the whole thing would be over? Maybe it wouldn't accomplish anything physically. But if it were some sort of pigeon placebo, more about faith than anything else, then I needed more than a bird. I still needed to find genuine faith, which was something I couldn't buy at a pet store.

# 14

# Ray of Light

MARCH 2006

I convinced Sam and Kimmi to sign up for an Omega conference being held at a hotel in Midtown in New York City. I'd never been to Omega's upstate campus in Rhinebeck, New York, and I longed to go to this center that offered programs on health, relationships, community, and "awakening the best in the human spirit." When I saw the title of this event, I knew I had to sign up: "Being Fearless." The mission, according to the brochure: "Unleash your own fearless spirit . . . Reinvigorate your purpose and passion for life. Delight in the surprise of fresh insights. Grow in strength and wisdom." On the roster were Jon Kabat-Zinn, Elizabeth Lesser, Gabrielle Roth, Byron Katie, Brian Weiss, Martha Beck, Debbie Ford, Iyanla Vanzant—the self-help all-stars. It had to be worth four hundred dollars a person.

Wayne Dyer and Caroline Myss spoke in the morning. I attended a breakout session with psychic James Van Praagh called

"Heaven & Earth: Making the Psychic Connection." I kept hoping my mom would pop up and say hello, but she didn't. There were crystals and tie-dye aplenty to buy in the gift center. Just as we were about to split, the buzz was that we had to get in to see this Zen master named Genpo Roshi. I didn't know much about Zen Buddhism, just that it was an ancient movement that encouraged meditation on the road to enlightenment.

I grabbed Sam and we went back inside. The class had already started. At first I was confused. The guy onstage looked Jewish, even though he was wearing a robe. Ah, it was the old Ram Dass/Prama thing. His name was Dennis Genpo Merzel Roshi. I would bet money that he was born Jewish but went Buddhist later in life. A Jew-Bu. It's not uncommon. (Indeed, he was born in Brooklyn, a descendent of a long line of Rebbes. He was ordained as a Zen monk in 1973.)

The core of his teaching is "the unshakable and contagious certainty that every one of us, regardless of our socioeconomic, cultural or religious background, can instantly awaken to our true nature, like the great masters of old — like the historical Buddha himself, whose essential teaching was nothing less than this. This experience helps us shed anxiety and fear and learn to live more purposeful, compassionate and joyful lives." As we entered, Genpo was describing a concept that he called "Big Mind" (this is a simplifed explanation of a complex concept, but bear with me). "Big Mind" is the state of clarity and wisdom, and "Big Heart" is the compassion one pursues on the road to self-discovery and enlightenment. He felt that everyone was born with "a Buddha mind," and that by taking Buddhist principles and infusing them with Western psychological terms (there's that balance thing again), it would spread Zen teachings rather than limit them to a bunch of dudes with shaved heads and yellow robes on a mountaintop. He called it "Western Zen." Genpo theorized that the Self could be broken down into various aspects or voices, and he had a whole list of these. "I'm going to ask to speak to a couple aspects of mind," he explained. "And I'll ask you to shift your posture between each. First, I'd like to speak to the Controller. What does the Controller do?" Genpo asked us.

People murmured, "He's in charge." "Takes care of everything." Sam raised an eyebrow at me. Eventually someone answered, "Controls."

Yep. "What does the Skeptic do?" Doubts. "What does the Protector do?" Protects. "What does the Vulnerable Child do?" Gets hurt . . .

I was starting to understand. Sure, there was a Damaged Child in me, but also a Protector. When you dissected these different voices, you could experience a stronger sense of self. It was an intellectual interpretation of Alora's theory that the "self" was made up of different organs and systems that each had a voice. I was the CEO of my body. I had to communicate with all these entities reporting to me to help my body run more efficiently on the way to wellness or Oneness.

Genpo Roshi walked us through his list, asking to talk to the Mind of Desire, then the Mind That Seeks "the Way." Finally, he requested an audience with "the Way."

If the Controller was part of me, and the Damaged Self, and I was those things . . . then inside myself I'd also find "the Way."

"What does the Way do?" he asked.

Someone in the crowd said, "Uh, it just is. It's just the Way, being the Way. Being."

*I am the Way.*

Ding ding! I felt this warm honey feeling grow in me and start to spread around the room. A flash, just a teeny one, of enlightenment. I get it: *I'm the Way. Sam is the Way. You are the Way. We are all the Way, and we are the same.*

I called Meghan (who is most definitely the Way) to recount this Big Mind process. Another friend from the University of Michigan days, she planned a women's circle of love when I got sick, inviting a group of my closest friends over to her place in the West Village to gather around me and fill me with positive energy. When my hair fell out, Meghan bought me a gorgeous Lulu Guinness silk head scarf, and wore one of her own in solidarity. I later dragged her to a Genpo session in New York. Her take on the Zen master? "He's sexy!" True. He was a pretty sexy monk. Meghan later sent me a section of a Gnostic poem about the nature of the feminine divine called "The Thunder—Perfect Mind" that resonated big time:

*I am the first and the last.*
*I am the honored one and the scorned one.*
*I am the whore, and the holy one.*
*I am the wife and the virgin.*
*I am the mother and the daughter. . . .*
*I am she whose wedding is great,*
*and I have not taken husband . . .*

*I am knowledge, and ignorance*
*I am strength, and I am fear.**

Wow, I am all of those things. I'm definitely the Way.

---

APRIL 2006

As confident as I felt about my healing course of action, eventually my liver enzyme levels again began to creep in the wrong direction. During the era when Jenny Lynch predicted I'd be having a great spiritual awakening, all I could hear were the words of the Number One Liver Expert in the World. He'd been sure that I had autoimmune hepatitis; in other words, my own cells were causing my demise. He'd told me that I had to go back on serious steroids and chemo *or else.* I'd told him to give me six months to find some alternative, promising that if I didn't I would follow his every directive. Number One's response?

"You don't have six months."

I asked Turner for his advice. Here I'd had this great alternative run, but I was hitting a standstill. Should I go back on serious medication? He said, "You've always made sound decisions about your medical care. But if you were my sister, I'd tell you to do the

* "The Thunder, Perfect Mind," from *The Nag Hammadi Library*, James M. Robinson, General Editor. Copyright 1978, 1988 by E. J. Brill, Leiden, the Netherlands.

chemo." Note: Whenever a doctor prefaces his opinion with the phrase "If you were my sister/mother/daughter/wife," he means business. So I took the drugs.

Within two days I knew I'd made the wrong decision; by losing faith in my choices, I'd betrayed myself and disrespected the wishes of my body. My system suffered way worse than any other times I'd gone through treatment. I launched into instantaneous steroid mania and stopped sleeping. My liver swelled so badly that I could literally see it straining out of my torso, like the monster in *Alien*. I was in so much stomach pain that I couldn't eat, and didn't want to, since I was pissing and shitting blood.

I returned to Miami for Passover with my family on a Thursday night in April. I got in an inane fight over the war in Iraq with Mick and Josh. I went to my hotel room and cried my eyes out to Carrie on the phone. Lying on the hotel bathroom floor in the middle of that night, in a cold sweat, immobilized from head and stomach pain, in steroid-induced psychosis, bleeding from various holes and fissures in my body (nose, gums, tear ducts, urethra, ass, and just as a little added F-U, I got my period as well), I gave up. I told Bigger Than Phil, "I would rather die than live like this." It was like the end of a movie, where some angelic presence is gesturing toward the heroine to come, come to the light. Only there was no light, and no was inviting me to drop by. I was basically knocking at the door and saying, "Lemme in, I'm ready to go!" And then I died.

But . . . not really. No spectral energy took me up on my offer to cross over. When the sun rose on Friday morning, my body rose, too (at the time, I didn't know it was actually Good Friday).

My nose stopped bleeding. Now I felt sort of half alive, half not. I left the hotel without speaking to anyone. I walked past the restaurant by the pool on the way to the beach, where a guy hosed down the tiles and sang: *"Don't worry about a thing....Every little thing's gonna be all right...."*

I walked south on the beach boardwalk and then cut into the city streets. When I could no longer walk, I sat at the News Café on South Beach. I was finally hungry. I ate scrambled eggs and a little bit of bagel. Yes, it was Passover, but I figured since I was already dead, a few carbs weren't gonna matter. I read the *New York Times* (MORE RETIRED GENERALS CALL FOR RUMSFELD'S RESIGNATION) and the *New York Post* (ISRAEL IN CRISIS OVER MADONNA!) cover to cover.

I called Turner to tell him I'd decided to stop all medication. In my expert opinion—and I had the sneaking suspicion that I, indeed, was an expert on my own body—the meds weren't fighting Wegener's; they were fighting symptoms and side effects. It was time to stop treating symptoms and start treating the root cause of the disease, whatever it may be. Turner was out of the office. I called Number One to tell him that I'd decided to stop all medication. He didn't call me back.

I took a cab back to the hotel in time for Shabbat dinner with my family. I freaked them out because I didn't eat a thing (in Jewish families, not eating is a terrible sign). On Friday night I went to sleep. On Saturday I woke up again. I felt a little better. By Sunday I was strong enough to fly back to New York. Josh helped me inch through the airport. I still felt like a ghost, but no one could tell.

Back home on Monday, I took lab tests. The lab was so horrified by the results on the liver enzymes that they called Number One to tell him my liver was failing. His assistant phoned me and explained, "There has to be an error. You need to retake the tests."

"Can I speak to the doctor, please?"

"He's busy."

Yeah? I'm busy dying.

I started dialing the names listed on the office contact sheet; everyone from the receptionist to the lab assistants got hit with a huge scary outburst from the eye of Storm Wendy. By the time Number One called back, I was emotionally and physically cashed. I crashed on a couch in Sam's Midtown office, which was down the street from the lab. I had no rage left to muster.

Over the phone he insisted, "You have to restart the medication."

"I'm not going to."

"Fine, then I will have to disavow you of medical care, and I won't expect to see you again."

I rolled my exhausted eyes at Sam. "You don't have to worry about it."

On Tuesday, I retook the labs. On Wednesday, they came back 50 percent better than they had been on Monday. I took them again a week later. Fifty percent improvement once again.

A week later, I went to Madonna's Confessions on a Dance Floor tour at Madison Square Garden. I danced with a fervor I'd never experienced before. I felt so powerful, so grateful to be in a body that was strong enough to twirl around, and generous enough to give me another chance. Madonna started performing my favorite song, "Ray of Light," and I sang along. We were revving up to the chorus: "*She's got herself a little piece of heaven, waiting for the time when earth shall be as ooooone . . .*"

And I feel! That's when I literally saw the Ray of Light. Right at the climax of the song, I hit the spiritual jackpot. The expanse of Madison Square Garden, every seat in the house, glowed with golden light. Kundalini energy zipped up my spine and burst straight out of my crown chakra. It was the same energy I'd felt on the chromatherapy table in Albuquerque that first time, times a thousand. Angels sang. The Way that Genpo Roshi had described revealed itself as a golden glow spread over the entire audience. It was *gu* and *ru* home run: darkness revealing light, ignorance defeated by ultimate knowledge. The long-blond-curly-haired goddess of Kabbalah had tapped me on the head, anointing me with her Madonna/Mary/Mother energy. I had the power to light up Madison Square Garden, and indeed the whole wide world, because I believed. I had faith.

Faith in what? Well, let's not get too specific. I didn't know what. It didn't matter. I just knew that I wasn't going anywhere. It was a phenomenal sensation, and I finally understood why the believers believed. I hadn't felt that kind of power in a long time, if ever. I am the Light. We are all the Light. Details . . . um, TBD.

Jenny Lynch had told me that a feeling of deep spiritual search and connection was going to start in March 2006. That was when

I stopped taking the meds. Now I knew my life's purpose, if not the details of how it was to unfold: I was ready, willing, and able to help illuminate the way for those who were lost in the dark.

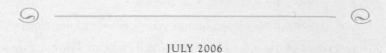

JULY 2006

July Fourth was a hot and festive day in New York City. Josh was throwing a party at his place so we could go up on the roof and watch the fireworks over the East River. Mick was in town and staying at a hotel in Columbus Circle. I was rollin' so high on the previous night's Madonna show that I couldn't eat or sleep.

On my way over to Mick's hotel, I got a call from Meghan on my cell. Just that day, she had broken up with her live-in boy-friend. While I hated to think of her suffering, I thought the split was perfectly timed. It was Independence Day for America, and Independence Day for Meghan, too. I knew she was in pain, but I also sensed that somehow the universe would take care of her. I was feeling really pro-universe in those days.

I ran around with my dad for a whole sweaty day. We finally ended up at Josh's apartment, where Mick enjoyed a few drinks before the fireworks began. I encouraged Meghan to join us down-town, hoping the spectacle would be a distraction, if not an in-spiration. They were. After the show, we wandered around the Financial District with thousands of other New Yorkers and tour-ists, not a cab to be found. Mick refused to get stranded on a hot, crowded subway platform. While he hunted for a ride, Meghan and I walked over to Ground Zero. Five years after 9/11, it still looked like an atomic crater surrounded by chain-link fence. I approached the fence and peered in, my heart breaking over all the pain that still lived there. I closed my eyes and sent out a little prayer to the families who had lost members there, and to all of us who had lost a kind of innocence and arrogance when they died. Mick shouted to us—he'd found a car.

I hopped into the backseat of a big-ass SUV, the kind that rental car companies use to shuttle clients to and from the airport. Mick and Meghan were already inside. In the driver's seat was a big black guy who had a sleeve of CDs tucked in the visor above his head. I couldn't tell if he was a professional chauffeur who had decided to take one extra fare for the night, or just some dude who had been driving when he saw my dad waving money in the air. Next to him in the passenger seat was a cute little kid, maybe five or six years old, with a DVD player in his lap. He was watching the tail end of *Bad Boys II* with Martin Lawrence and Will Smith. I thought the movie was too R-rated for a six-year-old to be watching, but then again, said six-year-old was driving around with his dad picking up randoms in their car at about midnight on a Wednesday. So maybe rules weren't the kid's strong suit.

"Meghan," asked Mick, "where do we drop you off?"

"You can go to Hudson and Tenth Street."

"Hey, chief," Mick called into the front seat. "Hudson and Tenth." We headed uptown on the West Side Highway. Mick tossed out the term *chief* in a way that made me wonder if the driver had introduced himself as "Chief," or if my dad had just given him that jovial appellation on a whim. While Mick and Meghan chatted about trends in women's footwear ("Why are some men so fascinated by high-heeled shoes?"), I tilted forward to the little boy in the passenger seat. Credits were running down the screen of his DVD player. "How ya doin'?" I asked. He just smiled. "Did you get to see the fireworks?" He shrugged. I could hear words like *arch* and *stiletto* being bandied around in the backseat. I asked the kid, "It's kind of late for you to be out, right?"

The chief just laughed. "Oh yeah, his momma's gonna kill me."

"I want to see another movie," the kid piped in.

"Which one?" the chief asked.

"Mmm, *Shark Tale*."

The chief plucked a DVD from the sleeve and handed it off to the kid, who popped it in the machine. I asked him, "So what's your name?"

Just then the chief pulled over to let Meghan out of the car. I was satisfied; we'd turned her potentially insufferable night around. In the front seat, the opening credits started to roll on the new movie. Animated, a lot of fish. The opening song began to play, and the kid bounced along to it: *Don't worry about a thing, every little thing's gonna be all right....*

I couldn't believe it was here again, this Bob Marley song called "Three Little Birds," like the three little birds who sat outside Alora's window. I felt some God-ish bumps creeping up my spine. "You know that song?" I asked the kid. No response. "It's got a pretty good message, right?"

The SUV pulled up in front of Mick's hotel and he hopped out. "Hey, chief!" he shouted. "Take care of my baby girl!"

"Will do," said the chief cheerfully. As the door slammed shut and the chief drove a few blocks uptown, I wondered for a moment if it was completely safe for my dad to have given some guy who may or may not be an official chauffeur a stack of cash and let him zoom away with me in the backseat. But I wasn't going to worry about a thing; God had just let me know he had my back by playing that song. The chief pulled up to my corner and I hopped out. "Happy Independence Day!" I called to him and his boy, but they were already driving away.

The next morning I was exhausted from the late night, but had to rise early to make my acupuncture appointment with Dr. Lipman. I took the subway downtown, hopped out at Twenty-third Street and Seventh Avenue, and rushed east on Twenty-second Street. The light flashed DON'T WALK and even though I was late, I hesitated on the corner. Next to me was an African-American woman clutching a boy by the arm. He was cute, about five or six years old. I did a double take. It was the boy from the car. The chief's son from the night before. Wait, how could that be? I must have been confused. But I could have sworn he was the same kid. "Hey," I said to him, "I know you!"

His mom glared at me. How on earth would some Manhattan girly-girl know her baby boy?

"From last night," I continued. "Do you remember? Driving in the car with your dad?"

"What are you talking about? He wasn't driving in no car." The mother crouched down to face the little boy. "Were you in a car last night with your father? I'm gonna kill that man! He was supposed to come with me today to buy this bed for you, but if you were running out with him last night . . ." The light changed and she began to yank the little boy across the street. But not before he turned around, looked at me, and began to sing, "Don't worry about a thing...Every little thing's gonna be all right."

Make sense of this, I ordered my brain. That couldn't possibly have been the same kid. Maybe I'm a racist and I think all six-year-old black boys look the same. Plus that song was from a kiddie movie. Maybe all kids his age know that movie . . .

Dr. Lipman gently poked me full of holes with his acupuncture needles and left me in the darkened room to simmer. I twisted my head out of the earphones that were gushing what were supposed to be soothing ocean sounds into my head. I needed to hear myself think. Then it hit me. Maybe that little boy was, like . . . a messenger from GOD.

I was pretty sure God wasn't some big old hairy white guy in a dress. And the idea that God was transferable made perfect sense. God, angel, messenger, Phil, whatever. God was in everyone, we were all the Way, and he had shown up in that little boy to give me a wink and let me know that everything was going to be just fine. I blissed out in peace on the table. Later that night, I went to dinner at an Ayurvedic restaurant on the Upper West Side with my friend Bonnie. I had also turned her on to Turner; she had suffered from lupus since she was a little girl. Hyped up on prednisone, we loved to plow through meals together. Once she looked around at our empty plates and sighed, "It's such a pleasure to eat with someone else who is on steroids." I wasn't a bit surprised when we walked up to the restaurant and saw a message written on the "specials" board: DON'T WORRY—EVERYTHING'S GOING TO BE ALL RIGHT.

Joe and I flew to see another Madonna show on July 9 in Boston. Best one yet. This time the transcendent moment hit me during "Jump": *Are you ready to jump? Don't ever look back, oh baby . . .* I was ready to jump, finally prepared to take a true leap of faith.

On the train ride home from Kennedy Airport, I read Caroline Myss's *Sacred Contracts*, a guide to Jungian personality archetypes. She theorized that if you could assess your archetypes, you could figure out your life's calling. Out of nowhere, or maybe from deep inside myself, I heard a voice. The "Let go" voice. I was pretty sure it was God.

God asked, "Would you be willing to come back to life fulltime?"

*Well, BTP, I'd like to, but . . .*

"No guarantees," God warned me. "It won't necessarily be a long life, or a healthy life, or an easy life, but it will be worth it."

By the time I transferred to the subway uptown from Penn Station, I was convulsing and shaking. Other straphangers shook their heads and moved away from me, as jaded New Yorkers usually do. I told God, Yes. And so, I was reborn.

# 15

# Like a Prayer

I once received a voice mail message on my home phone at 5 p.m. on a Friday from an office assistant at a radiology lab. Why she didn't dial my cell is anyone's guess. "Um, hi, this is _____ at _____ Clinic. Wow, the doctor really needs to talk to you. I guess we'll just try you back on Monday." Are you shitting me? That was easily one of the longest weekends of my life. See, a doctor is only as good as the weakest link on her office staff. The world's most brilliant physician can treat you, but if she can't find your chart, you're screwed.

Sick and tired (literally) and ridden with anxiety about some brain scan results that still hadn't surfaced as promised, I decided to hold my own private sit-in at a doctor's office. You know the story: "We'll have the results for you in five to seven days." It's all you can do to wait until day five. Nothing. Then it's the weekend. Next Monday you still haven't heard a thing. By now you've convinced yourself that you have an inoperable brain tumor and you start making plans to see the Pyramids and eat as much chocolate cake as you can before you die. Every day you're on the phone with the doctor's staff, until the receptionist has most certainly blown you off and put you on some sort of "Do Not Call This Psycho Back" list.

Finally the doctor left me a message assuring me there was nothing to worry about, but guess what? It was my *brain* we were waiting on. My brain was *worried*. Maybe in *his* brain all was well, but it wasn't so in *my* brain, the brain that had been scanned *two weeks* ago. At that point I wasn't nearly as worried about a brain tumor as I was about my head exploding from pure, unadulterated fury. So on a Monday morning, I packed up my computer, my briefcase, two newspapers, a bottle of water, and a cup of coffee. I showed up at the doctor's office at 8:30 a.m., spread all of my stuff out over seats in the waiting room, and informed the receptionist, "I will not leave until I receive the results from my test."

Apparently this doesn't happen a lot.

The staff flipped. An assistant came out to the waiting room and pledged, "The results will be fine. Go home. We'll contact you as soon as we can." I pledged right back, "I will not leave this office until I have results in my hand and I'm completely satisfied." I never lost my cool. I was as courteous as an infuriated patient with a possible brain tumor could be. When my doctor arrived he was informed of my sit-in. He guaranteed me once again, "Things are perfectly okay. When I get the results I'll call you right away. You can go home."

"I'm fine where I am."

Other patients in the waiting room were starting to notice trouble developing. The office manager approached me and suggested, "Why don't you move your stuff into the conference room where you can work with fewer disturbances?"

"Sounds like a great idea," I chirped.

A few minutes later another assistant poked her head in and said, "We need this conference room for a conference."

"Go ahead and confer; you won't bother me," I said brightly. While they eyed me nervously, a runner was finally sent to the X-ray center to personally pick up a copy of the results and bring them back to me. My doctor entered the conference room and handed me proof that there was nothing to worry my pretty little head about. Everything was fine. I thanked him, packed my stuff up, left, and never went back to his office again.

Maybe I was being irrational. But I had to take a stand. Business in a medical setting is not business as usual, especially when your well-being is the business at hand. If there was anything I knew with certainty, it was that my opinion about what was happening with my body was just as valuable as any doctor's.

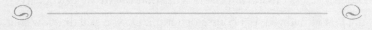

AUGUST 2006

Early on a sultry morning on the first day of August, I returned to see the Number One liver doc. I'd felt no urge to speak to him again; but Turner told me he'd called him repeatedly, voicing his concern about my well-being and his confusion about my disappearance from his appointment schedule. Turner begged me to make a follow-up appointment. Against my better judgment, I did.

Number One entered the room, smiled at me, and sat down.

He looked at my chart, flipped through the numbers, and folded it closed. "H.M." was scrawled on the front in marker. (I assumed they stood for "High Maintenance." That or "Her Majesty." Ooh, Her Madgesty!) In a tone cold enough to chill water to a temperature I no longer drank, he said, "I suppose you must feel rather vindicated about this whole situation."

"Vindicated?" I repeated. That wasn't necessarily the response I'd been expecting. "It's more like I feel grateful to be alive."

"No," he said firmly, eyes focused only on the folder. "You maintained that it was medication that was making you sick, and here are numbers that substantiate your theory. So I'm suggesting that you must feel quite vindicated about this whole thing."

"It's not really an issue of vindication," I told him. "Not really a win/lose. It's more about survival—"

He continued, "The last time we spoke on the phone, I suggested that you follow a prophylactic course of medication in order to stave off any adverse effects that might affect your liver, but you disavowed that course of action. Do you still disavow that course of action?"

*What is this?* I wondered. *An SAT test?* Hey, I sucked at the math, but I rocked the verbal. You can't use words to beat me at my own game, Doc; words are *my* weapons. I took a breath. "You would be hard-pressed to convince me to—"

"You said you disavowed that course of action. Do you still disavow that course of action?"

"Yes, I do."

"Fine. Then I will assume that your choice is not to pursue treatment."

"Oh, I'm pursuing treatment," I said. "It's just not what you'd recommend."

"What kind of treatment is this?"

"Body work. Ayurveda. Craniosacral therapy. Yoga. Meditation. Acupuncture. Anti-inflammatory vitamins and supplements—"

"Do any of these vitamins or supplements have names in a language that I would understand?"

"I don't know," I snapped. "Do you understand the name 'alpha-lipoic acid'?"

He put away the folder and rose from the desk. "Very well," he said. "I suggest you make an appointment to follow up with me in oh, four or five months or so. You should also get vaccinated for hepatitis A and hepatitis B. Let's hope I don't have to see you before then."

"Don't worry," I said. "You won't have to."

If docs were dates, this guy would have clearly won Bad Boyfriend of the Year. I left his office and walked out into the clear hot morning light of New York City, my adopted home. I recalled one of the songs that had elated me on Madonna's latest album: *"No other city ever made me glad except New York. . . . I love New York. . . ."*

I wasn't even mad at Number One; I felt sorry for him. I'd pulled down the curtain and exposed him as not a god but a regular, imperfect man who didn't have all the answers. He was so caught up in keeping score that he couldn't even say, "I'm glad you feel better." He may have been the world's leading expert on liver disease, but I was the world's leading expert on me. Sometimes Number One is really full of number two.

I went back to Turner's office later that week to take one more round of lab tests. I privately predicted that the results would show that my liver was healing, but my Wegener's had returned; I knew better than to think I could ever walk away with a completely clean bill of health. Turner was at his wits' end with me. He wanted me back on medication. Again I told him it was not an option. He cleared his throat and explained, "Sometimes . . . doctors have to let go of certain patients, even if they like and care about them."

"I'm sure that's true." I thought he was rationalizing Number One's attitude toward me. Only as I walked out of Turner's office did I realize he was breaking up with me.

The split didn't last long. Two days later, Turner reached me on my cell phone. "Are you sitting down?" It was like that call at the MTV studio all over again. But this time he told me with incredulity woven through his voice that the disease was gone and my liver was completely normal. "There's only one problem. The ANCA is way up. The Wegener's is back, but I'm not sure that medication is the answer. Maybe we should just get through this flare and reevaluate."

"I think that's a good idea," I gulped.

He hesitated. "The liver. I just . . . can't explain how this is medically possible."

I told him, "You don't have to."

I called Mick to give him the good news. He was so happy he started to cry. "You know it's HaShem, right?" he asked, using the Hebrew name for God. Well, I thought, according to Kabbalah God has seventy-two names, but . . .

"Yeah," I told him. "I know." Then I started bawling because he was, so hard that I gave myself a nosebleed. I was on the corner of Eighth Street and Sixth Avenue. Coincidentally (coincidences, another language God uses that I can understand), I was in front of the Barnes & Noble where I had done that first reading for *The Fat Girl's Guide to Life*, happy as can be and sick to death at the same time. I cried and hemorrhaged, feeling so incredibly relieved. I was four months away from my thirty-fifth birthday, and I was going to make it. Other New Yorkers shook their heads and stepped away from me, as jaded Manhattanites usually do.

*Oh, God,* I prayed. *Oh, HaShem. Oh, BTP. Oh Light, Oh Allah, Oh Goddess, Om Shanti, Oh, as Ricky Bobby would say, eight-pound, six-ounce, golden-fleeced, tiny baby Jesus. Thank you, thank you. I am so grateful. I'm also, um, a little bit confused. I'm not quite sure why I can't have complete health—why a clean liver and a functional immune system is too much to ask for at the same time, but I remember the terms of the Sacred Contract I signed with you on the train, on the way back from the Madonna concert in Boston. I signed on, without compromise. I will run on faith now, not fear. Still, a little clarification would be nice. A little more exposition, perhaps. Right now, how about if I go around the corner to the drugstore and buy myself some Kleenex?*

So there I was, standing in line at the Duane Reade drugstore above the godforsaken F-train subway entrance, with eyes full of tears and a face full of blood. The lady behind the counter was heavyset, had a lazy eye, and was taking her sweet-ass time ringing people up. I was doing the itchy, jumpy, New York City hurry-it-up-already-can't-you-see-I'm-in-trouble-here? dance, when I stopped myself: *Wendy Shanker, you just received what may arguably be the best phone call of your entire life. How 'bout you cut this rude behavior and thank your lucky star (ooh, "You may be my Lucky Star"?) and give this lady behind the counter a little bit of R-E-S-P-E-C-T? Because God only knows what she is going through in her life right now.*

I composed myself, focusing on the woman behind the register, and checked out her name tag:

BLESS D.

Okay, it wasn't "Blessed," like a complete verb. It was "Bless D.," as opposed to "Bless F." who might have been over in cosmetics, or "Bless P." who could have been counting stock in the back. However you want to read it, she was blessed in my book. My heart filled with love for my fellow woman as I pushed bloody little bundles of Kleenex and a Duane Reade discount card her way.

"Is that your real name?" I asked hesitantly.

"Mmm-hmm," she said, ringing me up.

"That's a pretty special name," I stuttered, smiling through my tears. I leaned in and whispered as if we had a secret code word, "Are you truly Blessed?"

She lifted her hands off the register, pushed my purchase back toward me with a receipt, tilted her head slightly down, locked her one good eye on me, and announced:

"*Next.*"

# CONCLUSION

## Into the Groove

H ere's the thing about having a chronic, incurable disease: it never ends. A few months after my illustrious spiritual awakening, I ended up in the hospital again. Just days before my thirty-fifth birthday. The news this time: I'd sprouted a bunch of fruit-sized (orange, peach, plum) granulomatous lung tumors. It was like bronchial fruit salad. Oh, so that explained why I'd barely been able to talk, or walk a block without pulling over and gasping for air. As proud as I was of my med-free decision, I had to go back on heavy doses of steroids and painkillers simply to survive. I consulted with one of Turner's associates at the Mayo Clinic in Rochester, Minnesota. He examined me, considered my options, and concluded with something along the lines of "Here's the way I see it. I am an expert in pulmonary issues of Wegener's granulomatosis. I can tell you about every study, every patient. I know everything medically. But you are the expert on you. So, what do you say we pool our resources and figure this out together?"

The magic words. The litmus test for all the doctors and healers I've worked with since that time: You're the expert on (fill in the blank). I'm the expert on me. Let's work together to make things better. Work with the mind in the middle.

The Mayo team and Turner felt strongly that continuing rounds of Rituxan would be the best course of action. So far, they're right. As of this writing, I've been off prednisone for eighteen months, and in clinical remission for at least six months. A brilliant ENT surgeon at Mayo repaired my nose by using cartilage and bone harvested from one of my ribs. I'm still seeing Dr. Turner, to whom I am forever indebted. I remain appreciative of Dr. Allen's care, but switched to an ENT with a gentler touch. After the liver team at Mayo finally and correctly diagnosed me with hepatitis C (not autoimmune, but viral, *hello*, and likely contracted during one of my medical procedures), I hooked up with a female hepatologist in New York. Upon our first examination she asked me, "Have you ever considered doing meditation? I don't know if it changes things medically, but I certainly believe it helps the body prepare itself for healing." East and West are moving closer together each day. For example, Donna Karan's Urban Zen Foundation is on a mission to "change the current healthcare paradigm to include integrative medicine and promote patient advocacy" with tools such as nutrition, yoga, and Eastern healing practices. I find more and more doctors who are interested in exploring these issues.

I often think back to Prama, who told me to find the middle place. I've tried to stop thinking of myself as healthy or sick. Good or bad. Fat or thin. Allopathic medicine or integrative healing. Physically, mentally, and spiritually I'm finally starting to understand that my road to enlightenment—especially around my issues of health, positive body image, and self-love—isn't just a switch that flicks on and off, like the lights hanging over the chromatherapy table at the Ayurvedic Institute. For example, I thought once I'd rectified my issues with my weight, I was done with the issue. At peace with my body. Yay! Completely enlightened. Then, just as the pounds had always come on against or despite my will, they dropped off due to my sick liver. Issue not over, thank you very much. As my friend Marta explained to me, "The Wendy who wanted to be a star and prove to the world that it was okay to be fat wound up with a much bigger issue: to prove to yourself that you needed to love your body enough to fix it, and trust yourself to make the right decisions."

Enlightenment isn't instantaneous. It's more like, when the light switch flips on, there's electricity running. Enlightenment is available, and now that you can see, you have to look for it. I'm sure, most definitively, that I saw "the light" at that Madonna concert. But I don't have auto-access to it when I need it. I thought that meant I'd missed my chance to be enlightened; the window opened, then slammed shut. Not the case. The opportunity remains. Now I'm starting to understand that the mission is not about seeing the light, but about searching for it.

Tracy recently introduced me to the teachings of a Zen teacher named Adyashanti, who explained this concept so thoughtfully in a writing called "An Inner Revolution":

The moment of awakening shows us what is ultimately true and real as well as revealing a deeper possibility in the way that life can be lived from an undivided and unconditioned state of being. But the moment of awakening does not guarantee this deeper possibility, as many who have experienced spiritual awakening can attest to. Awakening opens a door inside to a deep inner revolution, but in no way guarantees that it will take place."*

I met so many gurus, hoping they would have the Answer. Doctors told me to take medicine. Dr. Rai told me to forgive. The rabbi told me to have faith. Alora told me to talk to my body. Genpo told me to open my Big Mind. Jenny told me to treat my emotional wounds. Prama told me to find a middle place. And Madonna told me to be brilliant. "Go ahead," she said. "Be brilliant."

I thought by "brilliant" she meant I should be smart, or try to impress her. In that moment, maybe she did. But being brilliant also means radiating light. She gave me permission—or maybe she ordered me—to shine light. To be a ray thereof, as her song says. Now *that's* a guru. Maybe someday I'll be able to consistently shine away, but I have to keep searching for the light before I can begin to reflect it. Just as Madonna swings between poles of strength and vulnerability, I do too. Illness makes you vulnerable, whether you'd like to be or not. I keep reminding myself that it's okay—maybe even beneficial—to ask for help. Just as I don't expect a doctor to have all the answers, I need to acknowledge my own power in saying "I don't know." There's an opportunity for my

---

* Adyashanti, "An Inner Revolution," 2008.

thinking to change and evolve. Madonna reinvents herself all the time. So can I.

I will tell you what I tell myself: Thick or thin, healthy or sick, success is not simply a matter of will or effort. Sometimes your body is just your body, however it looks, whatever your attitude, with all its faults. You may not have the power to fix it, but you do have the ability to start healing yourself by making choices that help you. You know your body better than anyone else possibly could. When you assess what your (realistic) goals are for it, you can achieve them. Then you empower yourself by finding the doctors, healers, and supporters who are willing to help you on your personal mission. You are not a percentage point or a statistic. It doesn't matter if 99 percent of people get better when they take a certain drug—when you're the patient, the odds are always fifty-fifty: The drug or treatment will work, or it won't. If it doesn't, you move on to the next one. Sometimes one specific protocol doesn't do the trick. Or it succeeds for someone else, but not for you. Choose the best, most effective elements from all the options and decide what particular recipe works for you. Once you decide what you want to do, and who can help you to do it, a completely different kind of healing begins. (Even Gwyneth got her guru on, studying Kabbalah with Madge and creating her on-line "GOOP" lifestyle newsletter.) It took me years to figure that out, then a few more to actually believe it. I wrote this book to save you time and angst, whether you have an autoimmune disease or love someone who does. When asked to describe what she'd learned from Kabbalah, Madonna said, "We are all responsible for our actions, our behavior, and our words, and we must take responsibility for everything we say and do. When you get your head wrapped around that, you can no longer think of life as a series of random events—you participate in life in a way you didn't previously. I am the architect of my destiny. I am in charge. I bring that to me, or I push that away. You can no longer blame other people for things that happened to you."*

People talk about doctors having a God complex, and over the years I met plenty who thought they were superbeings who could decide my fate. But if not big-G Gods, they have to at least be godly for you to give your faith over to them and trust them to keep you alive and well. Many were brilliant, but lacked heart. I was lucky with my primary Wegener's team in particular. They had a level of sensitivity in addition to the confidence it takes to go into a career where you are in charge of someone's life or potential death—or at least their day-to-day comfort level. At my old MTV workplace, a big mistake was spelling "Janeane Garofalo" wrong. In a medical setting, a big mistake is a flatline during a routine exam. After you brush away parental pressure and a lifetime of watching *ER*, some flip of a switch in doctors-to-be must help them decide that they have the capability to help sick people feel better. Even me.

No single guru had all the answers. But I found that it was only when I rejected the idea that one person had all the answers

---

* Maureen Orth, "Madonna Unbowed, Uncowed, Still Taking on the World," *Vanity Fair*, May 2008.

that I actually began to find some. In a poem called "Enlightenment," Dr. Vasant Lad writes:

*Do not look outside yourself.*
*No one can enlighten you.*
*Even the guru is just a mirror.*\*

I saw my reflection. I'm not arrogant enough to consider myself a guru in the traditional sense, but when it comes to Wendy Shankerism, I am my own guru. My own Best Guy. I realized I could take an element from all those wise people, add my own expertise, and come up with a treatment plan. I may not find a cure, but I can try to find a new way to live. I can't believe I was so worried about becoming one of "those people"—the seekers, the searchers, the chanters. I realized it doesn't make me a hypocrite to borrow some ideas for healthy, less stressful living (another example of finding balance). I'm doing my best to stay open-minded. Jenny told me that once I healed my wound, I could teach others how to do it. So that's what I'm trying to do. And to tell you the truth . . .

I feel rather vindicated about the whole thing.

---

\* Vasant Lad, "Enlightenment," in *Strands of Eternity*.

# Acknowledgments

"I thought of all the times my friends have given off light in the darkness, by their generosity, by trying to help in the world, by simply making it through the hard patches with a little dignity, so that other people could see this could be done."

—Anne LaMott, *"The Binge from Hell (and Back),"* O, July 2006

Grateful thanks to:

My parents, Susie, Mickey, & Myrna;

My brother, Josh, and my aunt, Nancy Faith;

The Tracys, Boy and Girl, literary sages both;

The doctors, healers and their teams who've gotten me this far;

And all the friends, family and colleagues who supported me through this journey and the writing of this book with love, laughter, pep talks, constructive criticism, and fizzy beverages.

You have helped me keep, keep it together. *Namaste.*

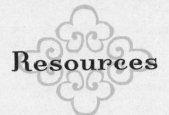

# Resources

VASCULITIS FOUNDATION
(WEGENER'S GRANULOMATOSIS)
P.O. Box 28660
Kansas City, MO 64188-8660
800-277-9474
816-436-8211
www.vasculitisfoundation.org
vf@vasculitisfoundation.org

ADVOCACY FOR PATIENTS WITH CHRONIC ILLNESS
Jennifer C. Jaff, Esq.
860-674-1370
www.advocacyforpatients.org
patient_advocate@sbcglobal.net

CLEVELAND CLINIC
800-223-2273
http://my.clevelandclinic.org

MAYO CLINIC
(Rochester, Minnesota)
507-538-3270
www.mayoclinic.com

DR. LOUIS J. ARONNE
CARDIOMETABOLIC SUPPORT NETWORK
1165 York Avenue
New York, NY 10065
212-583-1000
www.cmsnonline.com

THE AYURVEDIC INSTITUTE
11311 Menaul Blvd NE
Albuquerque, NM 87112-2438
505-291-9698
www.ayurveda.com

FRANK LIPMAN, MD
ELEVEN ELEVEN WELLNESS CENTER
32 West 22nd Street #5
New York, NY 10010
212-255-1800
www.drfranklipman.com

KRIPALU CENTER FOR YOGA & HEALTH
Stockbridge, Massachusetts
866-200-5203
www.kripalu.org

CHABAD LUBAVITCH
www.chabad.org

JENNY LYNCH, ASTROLOGER
www.jennylynch.com
dearjenny@jennylynch.com

THE UPLEDGER INSTITUTE, INC.
(CRANIOSACRAL THERAPY)
11211 Prosperity Farms Rd., Suite D-325
Palm Beach Gardens, FL 33410
561-622-4334
800-233-5880
www.upletdger.com
upledger@upledger.com

OMEGA INSTITUTE/"BEING FEARLESS"
150 Lake Drive
Rhinebeck, NY 12572
877-944-2002
845-266-4444
www.eomega.org

GENPO ROSHI/BIG MIND BIG HEART
1268 East South Temple
Salt Lake City, UT 84102
801-328-8414
www.bigmind.org
bigmindoffice@bigmind.org

OFFICIAL MADONNA WEB SITE
www.madonna.com

For blog, tours and other info about Wendy:
WENDY SHANKER
www.wendyshanker.com
wendy@wendyshanker.com
www.facebook.com/wendyshanker
http://twitter.com/wendyshanker

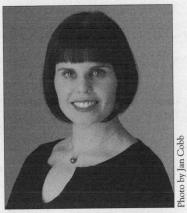

Photo by Jan Cobb

**Wendy Shanker**'s humorous, hopeful memoir about women and body image, *The Fat Girl's Guide to Life*, changed the way women around the world relate to their weight and bodies. It was published in ten languages including Italian, German, Spanish, Chinese, and Polish (but not French—because French women don't get fat). Wendy's work has appeared in *Glamour, Self, Shape, Cosmopolitan, Us Weekly*'s Fashion Police, alternative mags like *Bust* and *Bitch*, and on MTV, Oxygen, and Lifetime. Her essays can be found in *The Modern Jewish Girl's Guide to Guilt; Sex, Drugs & Gefilte Fish: The Heeb Storytelling Collection*; and *Does This Book Make Me Look Fat? Stories About Loving—and Loathing—Your Body*. This is her second book.